Helping Through
Illness

Practical Ways to Support Someone
with a Serious or Chronic Condition

Sheila Hoover

HERON SPRING PRESS

For Kat

Contents

Introduction

People with serious or chronic health conditions need practical support and tender loving care. Unfortunately, our society doesn't teach us how to provide this type of care, and figuring out how to help or what to say can be daunting. That's where this book comes in handy, because helping each other is what makes the world work. Oftentimes we operate under the illusion that there is an "us" (healthy) and a "them" (sick). The reality is that we will all be called on to help others at some point in our lives, and we will all need help ourselves.

Helping Through Illness contains dozens of concise, practical tips for supporting someone with a serious illness or chronic health condition, whether you are a family member, friend, neighbor, coworker, or acquaintance. In this book, the meaning of "support" includes anything from giving a grocery gift card to being an advocate in the health-care system. This book will quickly teach you:

- How best to help
- What to say (and not say)
- How to be sensitive to the person you're supporting
- How to take care of yourself while providing support

Helping Through Illness lightens a heavy topic by pairing each tip with an amusing cartoon featuring the main character, Ailey Cat, and their Care Cat friends. It was challenging to come up with a name for a cartoon cat who represents someone with a serious or chronic illness, because there are no good words in the English language to describe someone who is ill. Words such as "sick," "infirm," "invalid," and others sound negative. They also don't work to refer to someone who is living with a chronic health condition but doesn't identify as being "sick." So, the character is named Ailey Cat, which feels like a more thoughtful way to refer to someone who is ailing.

Quickly scanning the table of contents will get you started. Then you can either open the book to any page or read it from cover to cover. The tips are intended to be read in any order. At the core of all these tips is being sensitive to someone who is suffering and showing up for them (and yourself) with kindness, respect, and compassion.

Every Ailey Cat and every situation is unique. Some Ailey Cats are ambulatory, some are bed-ridden. Some are in the early stages of an illness, some are in an advanced stage. Some have chronic health conditions that they must manage their entire lives. Given this broad range, your role may also take different forms (and evolve over time). You may be your Ailey Cat's primary Care Cat, responsible for managing and delivering most of their care. You may be on standby to offer help as needed. You may be offering occasional support from a distance. Whatever the situation and your level of involvement, know that any help you give is much appreciated, and that even small gestures can make a big difference.

At the same time, it's important to be discerning about the kind of support you can appropriately offer. For example, if you are not part of the Ailey Cat's inner circle, offering to be their emergency contact is likely off the table. Instead, gifting a subscription to a streaming service may be just the right thing. You'll find these tips and dozens more in this book; just consider how well you know the Ailey Cat before making an offer of help. A good rule of thumb is to ask your Ailey Cat (or their primary Care Cat) first if they want or need what you would like to offer.

Also note that this book provides tips for Ailey Cats who are living with a serious illness or chronic health condition. It doesn't cover end-of-life issues and care—that would be another book!

HOW I CAME TO WRITE THIS BOOK

After I wrote my first book, *Helping Through Heartache, an Easy Guide to Supporting Anyone Who Is Grieving,* featuring Sad Cat, my friends who either had or were caring for someone with a serious illness asked if I could write a similar book for them. The central theme of the Heartache book—which is how to be sensitive, kind, and supportive to someone who is grieving—resonated with them and their experiences.

This made me reflect on my own experiences helping several friends and family members who had different types of cancers, ALS, and chronic health conditions. I also took care of my late husband for many years prior to his passing. (He is the one who taught me how to "hold light" for him instead of worrying, which is one of the tips in this book. It was a profound practice for me and I hope you find it helpful, too.) I interviewed Ailey Cats with a variety of health challenges and saw that there are many shared (and often heartbreaking) stories across their experiences. These experiences helped shape the cartoons and reinforced what I know to be true—that a little sensitivity can go a long way.

THE GIFT OF HELPING SOMEONE
THROUGH THEIR ILLNESS

Providing support and care to someone can take a lot of time and energy. It can also be a gift. I don't want to paint an idealistic, unrealistic picture of Ailey Cats as paragons of grace in the midst of pain. Rather, I believe that when we make a gesture to help someone who is having a hard time, there is always rich potential to learn and grow ourselves. We can learn empathy and compassion. We can be reminded to be grateful and appreciate what's really important in life. We can learn patience.

Ailey Cats can serve as a mirror, reflecting back to us where we can evolve and cultivate more compassion and goodwill for others. We can learn about grace and humility in the face of great challenges. We can feel the power of holding space with someone in pain. We can learn about our own emotional strength and resilience, what it looks like to fall apart and dig deep and somehow manage to keep going. We can learn that it's okay to not be okay. And, perhaps most important, we can learn about surrender and radical acceptance in the face of things over which we have no control, and let that soften our hearts, humble us, and teach us love.

ADVOCATING FOR ALL AILEY CATS

In addition to supporting Ailey Cats on a personal level, advocating for health equity and accessibility on a broader societal level is very important. Some of our Ailey Cats are disproportionately affected by serious or chronic illness due to structural racism and systemic bias, and therefore have a greater need for more tender loving care and practical support. We can all do our part to advance health equity. A good place to start is by learning more about social determinants of health, health disparities, structural oppression, unconscious or implicit bias, and institutional racism, and then taking action either individually as an ally in your community and beyond, or by supporting the people and organizations who are working to advance health equity.

It's my hope that the tips offered here will make providing support less daunting, and that this book will make a positive difference in the life of someone who has a serious illness or chronic condition, even if it's just a little.

Simple Ways to
Help Your Ailey Cat

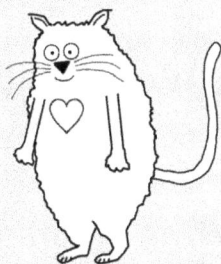

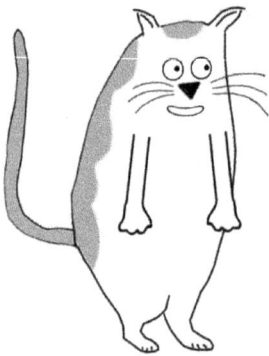

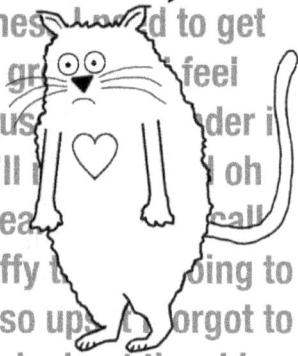

Give Your Ailey Cat a List of Specific Things You Can Do

People often say to an Ailey Cat, "Let me know if you need anything," and leave it at that. Ailey Cats, especially those who are in the midst of intense treatments, symptoms, or the demands of managing an unexpected and dramatic life change, may not have a clear sense of what they need. It may also be difficult for an Ailey Cat to reach out and ask for help, or to discern which offers of help are genuine.

Instead, make specific offers, such as, "I could run errands for you on Tuesdays." Look through the suggestions on the following pages for more ways to help. Then, give your Ailey Cat a list and say, "Here is a list of specific things I can do to help. I'm putting the list on the fridge. Call me if you need help with any of these things and I will show up."

If your Ailey Cat has other helpers, you could make this offer to them, too.

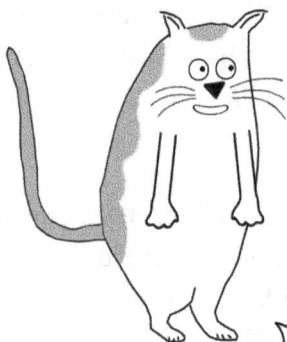

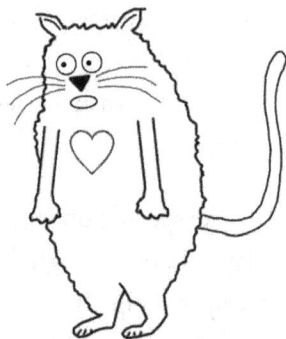

Check with Your Ailey Cat Before Jumping In to Help

Depending on the situation, it's usually better to check with your Ailey Cat (or their primary Care Cat, if they have one) before doing something you think is helpful. If your Ailey Cat says no to your offer, respect that. If they say "I'll let you know," that means *no* (at least until they get back to you).

If you can't get a clear yes or no, it may be because your Ailey Cat is distracted or struggling and can't process your request at that moment. Use your best, most sensitive judgment—if the task must be done right away, it may be best to just do it. If it's not that urgent, it may be best to wait until the Ailey Cat can give you a more definitive response.

It can be frustrating when you can clearly see that your Ailey Cat would benefit from a particular task getting done but they don't have the attention for it right then. Knowing when to lean in and when to step back is an art. You could say, "Okay, I'll leave [the task] for now but I'll keep an eye on things and check back in with you later."

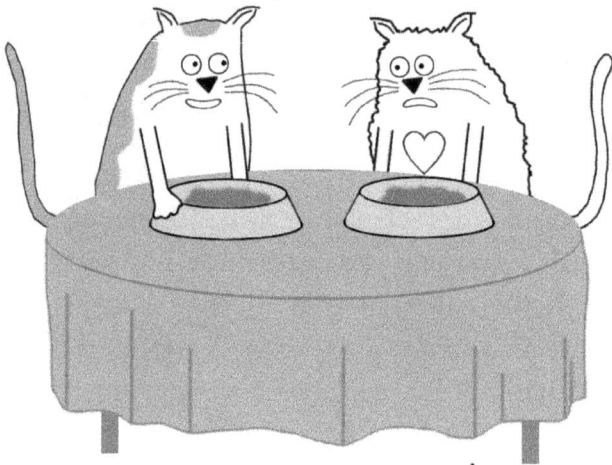

Has celiac disease, an autoimmune disorder that has no cure. It is not a food allergy or gluten sensitivity. Even traces of gluten can wreak havoc on their intestinal tract.

Help with Meals

Providing food can be a really great way to support your Ailey Cat. Check in with them first about what they would like to eat, and when. Remember to ask about any specific dietary needs and make sure you adhere to them exactly—what to you might seem like an insignificant divergence from their diet could lead to a lot of distress for your Ailey Cat.

Other ways to help with food are to:

- Organize a meal train (in consultation with your Ailey Cat) so everyone knows:
  - What type of food they need
  - How much food they need
  - How they would like it to be delivered (for example, left at the door so they don't have to get out of bed)
- Give restaurant or grocery-delivery gift cards
  - This allows the Ailey Cat the flexibility to use them as needed and to order the exact type of food they want.
  - If your Ailey Cat has children, it can be especially helpful to be able to use a gift card and make dinner happen without much effort.

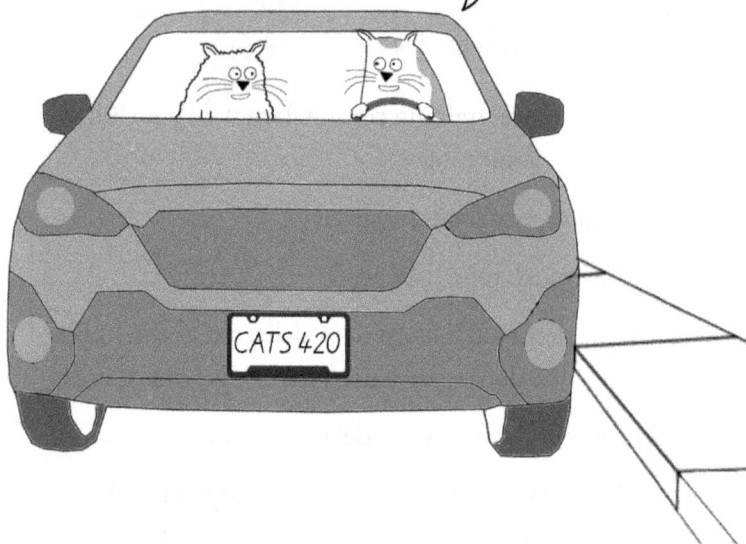

Give Rides

Giving your Ailey Cat a ride to appointments can be a great help. Getting dropped off at the door and picked up afterward can make a difficult appointment so much less stressful. Maybe stop for coffee on the way home.

You could also offer to run errands for your Ailey Cat or to be their chauffeur.

It's important to think through your Ailey Cat's needs and pre-solve any issues, especially if they have mobility challenges:

- Can they easily get in and out of your car?

- How far can they walk?

- Can you safely assist them?

- If they use a wheelchair, do you know how to operate and safely store it?

- Do they have a Disabled Person Parking Permit hangtag?

- Is the building accessible? (Does it have alternatives to stairs? Is the entryway wide enough?)

It can also be helpful to maintain your Ailey Cat's car, such as taking it in for oil changes, checking the tires, or washing it.

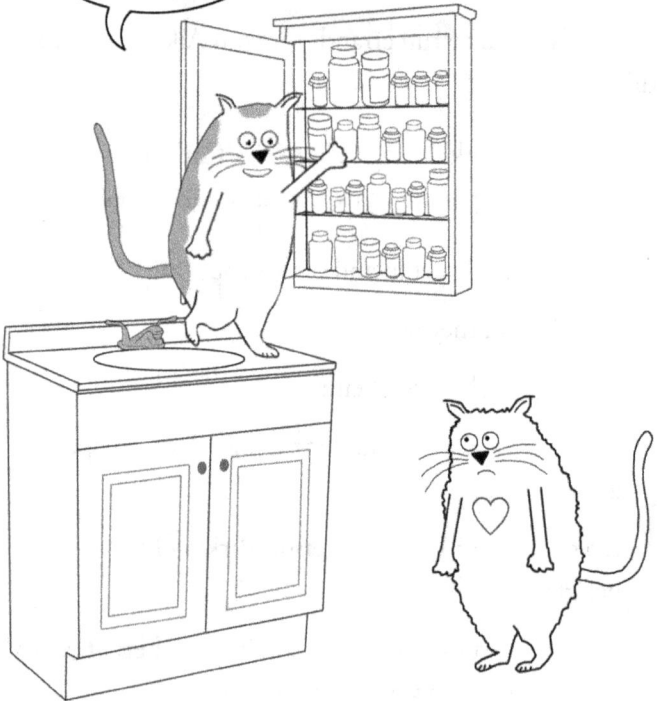

Clean Your Ailey Cat's Home

Cleaning your Ailey Cat's home can be really helpful, especially if it doesn't require too much energy on their part to provide direction. Some things to consider:

- Appreciate that having someone clean your personal space can make some people feel really vulnerable—ask if there are places they'd like you to leave as is.

- Ask your Ailey Cat if they need you to use certain kinds of cleaning supplies (scent-free, natural, etc.).

- Try to leave everything in the same place you found it, unless your specific task is to put things away.

- Ask your Ailey Cat if they are okay with you doing their laundry and if they have specific instructions to follow.

You could also hire a regular cleaning service for your Ailey Cat (if it doesn't stress them out too much to have someone they don't know in their space).

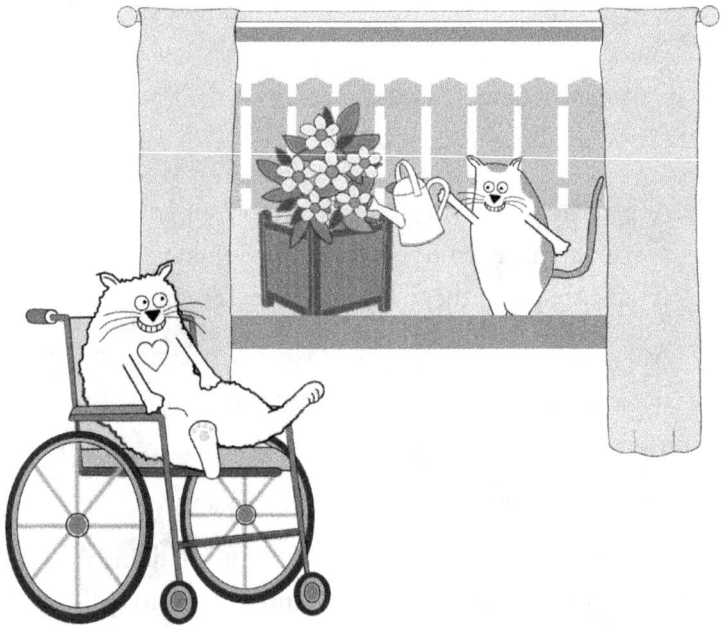

Do Yardwork

If your Ailey Cat lives in a house, you could offer to help with yardwork such as:

- Mowing the lawn regularly
- Cleaning the gutters as needed
- Tree maintenance
- Planting or maintaining a garden

You could also hire a yard service to provide ongoing maintenance.

If your Ailey Cat lives in an apartment, you could offer to regularly take care of any house plants.

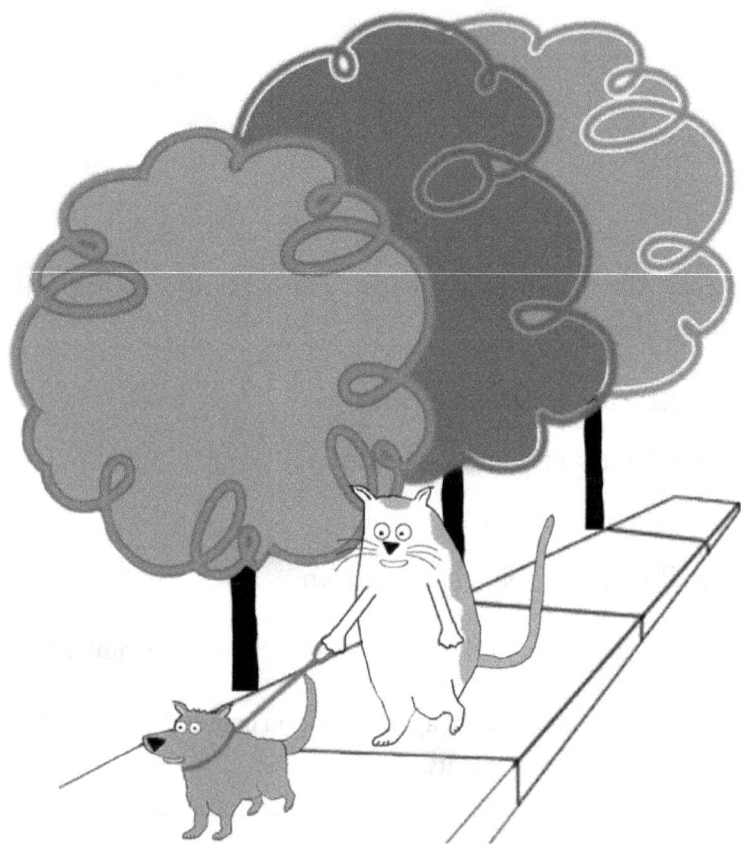

Help with Pets

Pets can be a great comfort to Ailey Cats, but they can also be a challenge to care for properly when their owner's health has been compromised. You could offer to:

- Take the pet for walks
- Play with the pet
- Clean a litterbox or crate
- Buy pet food or litter (or carry heavy bags)
- Take the pet to veterinary appointments or pay for their care
- Trim the pet's nails
- Pet-sit, if needed

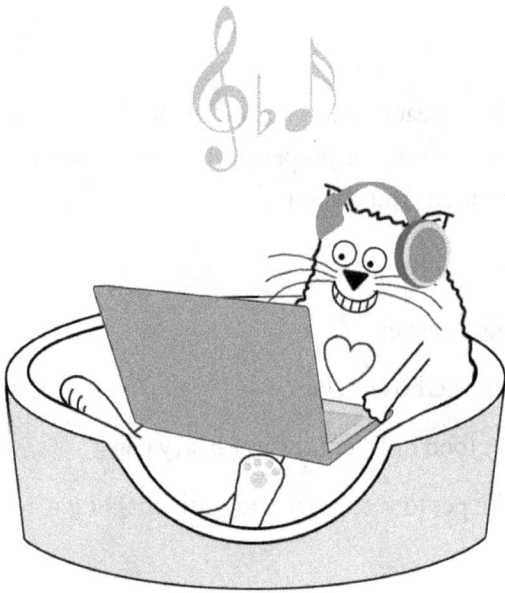

Give Subscriptions for Streaming Services, Books, or Magazines

A iley Cats may have a lot of down time waiting at doctors' offices, labs, or hospitals, or resting in bed. Gifting a subscription to popular movie or music streaming services, book clubs, or magazines can be a really nice gesture.

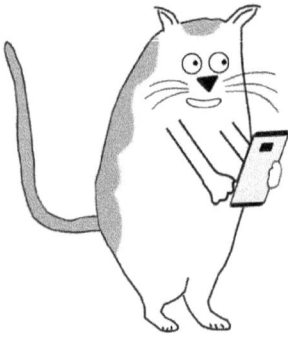

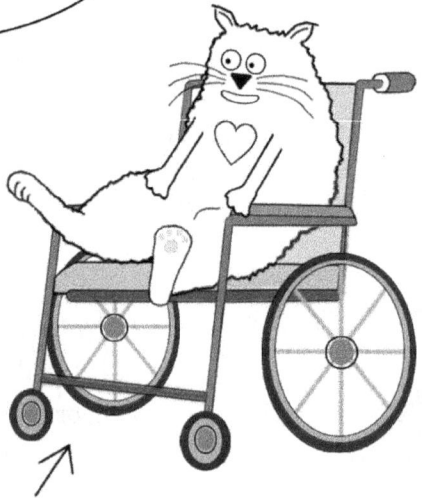

Contribute to Travel Expenses

I n some cases, Ailey Cats have to travel (sometimes far distances) to see specialists and receive treatment not available closer to home. For these Ailey Cats, it can make a big difference to receive help with traveling costs, including airfares (consider donating airline miles), food, lodging, rental cars, airport shuttles, medical supplies, and so on.

For Ailey Cats who are traveling alone, you could also help by:

- Giving them rides to and from the airport
- Arranging for a wheelchair upon arrival, if needed
- Accompanying them on the trip
- Helping to identify local support resources
- Shipping essentials to their destination so they don't have to carry them in their luggage

For Ailey Cats who must leave kittens at home, consider helping with childcare and communications between your Ailey Cat and their kittens.

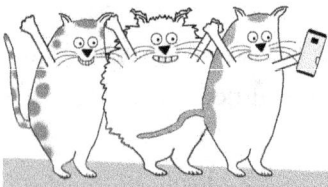

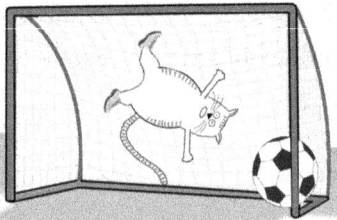

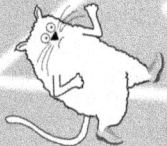

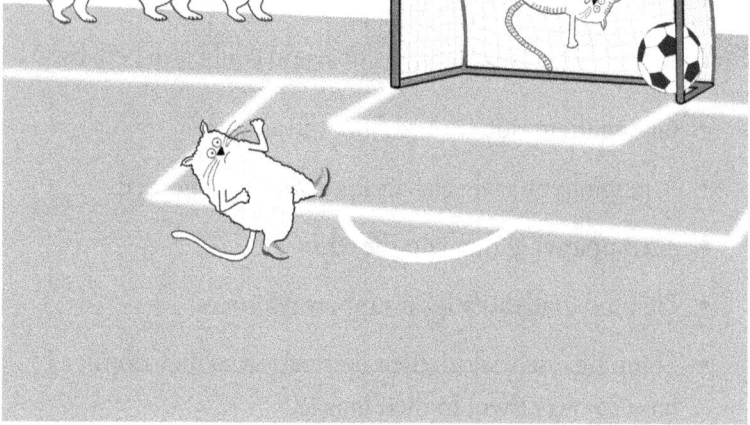

Film an Event for Your Ailey Cat and Show It to Them Later

t's really hard for Ailey Cats when they have to miss out on important events like birthdays, graduation ceremonies, kids' events, and weddings. You could offer to attend an event on their behalf and take photos or video to show them later.

Note that this requires sensitivity, as the idea of someone else being there when they cannot may be too painful. Respect your Ailey Cat's wishes if they decline your offer.

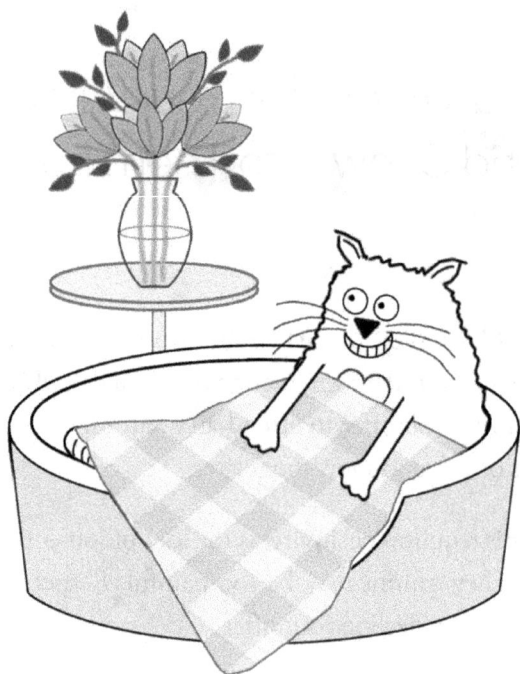

Beautify Your Ailey Cat's Environment

Having a soothing and aesthetically pleasing environment can be a great boost to an Ailey Cat. Sometimes, simple things can make a big difference—a bright new cushion or a beautiful plant, or always having a bouquet of fresh flowers on their table.

Ask your Ailey Cat if they would like help with that and in what way. Changing things in an Ailey Cat's environment requires a high level of sensitivity; for example, you don't want to burn incense that's too strong, or change colors to those they don't like, or rearrange their furniture in a way that doesn't work for them.

You could also put together a collection of special items on a table, such as photos of loved ones, special mementos, candles, sacred items from their religious or spiritual tradition, flowers, a string of lights, a tabletop water fountain, a beautiful tablecloth—whatever they would enjoy.

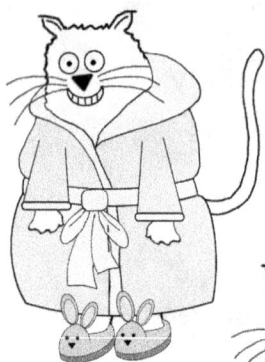

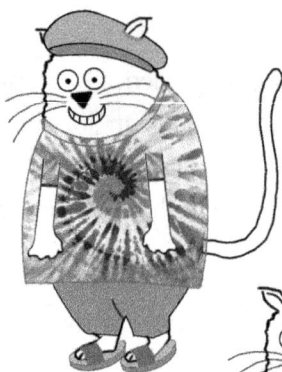

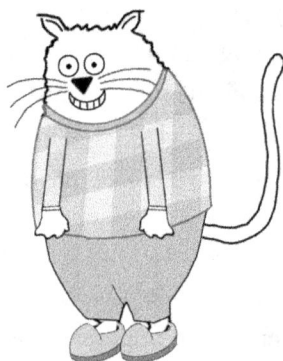

Give Your Ailey Cat
a Thoughtful Gift

Your Ailey Cat may really appreciate receiving a gift that provides comfort, beauty, or entertainment, or just cheers them up. Some ideas include:

- New clothes: Sometimes Ailey Cats' bodies change so much that none of their clothes fit. It can be a great boost to get some new clothing that reflects their personal style, or comfortable sweats or pajamas. You could help your Ailey Cat choose items online or give a gift card from their favorite place.

- A cozy throw or heated blanket

- Hats, scarves, or warm socks

- Satin pillowcases

- Self-care items such as Epsom salts or lotions (either unscented or their favorite scent)

- Snacks

- Books and magazines

- Herbal teas

- Small stuffed animal

- Items that say "I love you" (if appropriate)

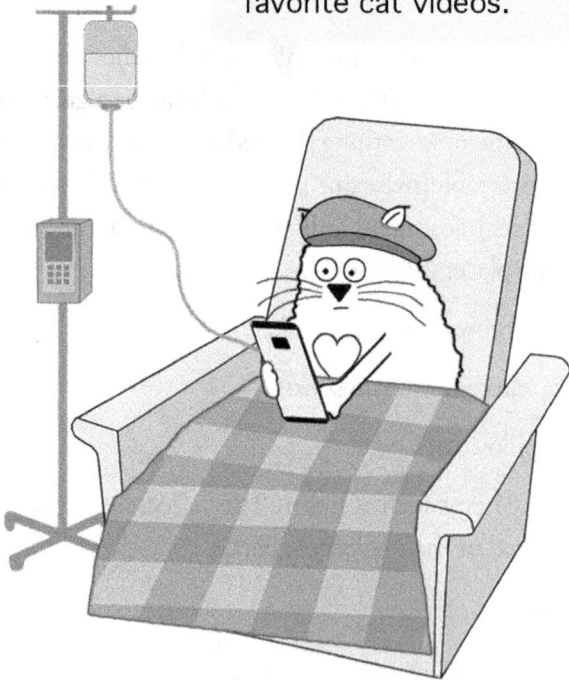

Support Your Ailey Cat's Social Connection

Dealing with a serious or chronic health condition can be very isolating, particularly for Ailey Cats who have been dealing with a chronic illness for a long time. It's important to keep in mind that Ailey Cats have no control over the ups and downs of their illness. They often don't know how they're going to feel day to day or even hour to hour. So, the connections with people who understand and can accommodate their need for flexibility become even more precious.

You can help support your Ailey Cat's social connection by:

- Reassuring them that they can be completely honest about how they're feeling, and that they don't have to pretend to be okay so as not to disappoint you

- Hanging in there over time and being flexible, even if it's frustrating when your Ailey Cat declines or cancels invitations at the last minute

- Following through on social occasions when your Ailey Cat does have the energy to show up

- Setting up an ongoing, regular social occasion with the caveat that your Ailey Cat can cancel if they wish, with no hard feelings

- Being a texting buddy—someone to whom your Ailey Cat can text simple things throughout their day; this can be especially helpful for Ailey Cats who live alone

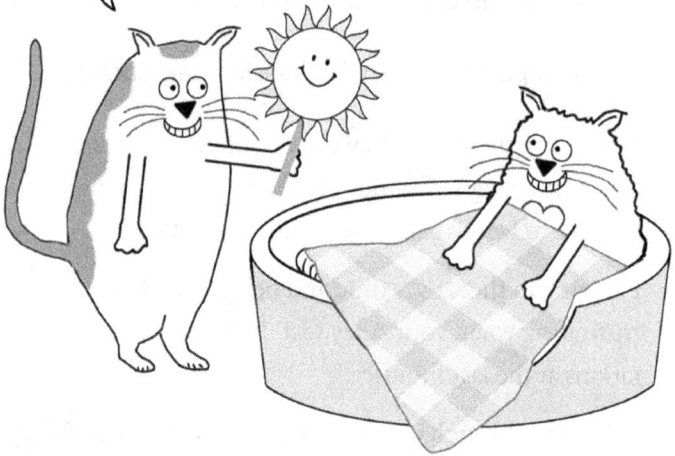

Celebrate Holidays with Your Ailey Cat

Holidays may be challenging for Ailey Cats, especially if they live alone. What used to feel like a happy celebration may be difficult given their health issues. Ailey Cats may not have the bandwidth to plan for holidays but may still enjoy doing something to acknowledge the day.

Ask your Ailey Cat what (if anything) they would like to do. If they would like to do something but can't think of anything, be prepared to offer some ideas. You could do something as simple as having a cup of tea while putting up decorations, watching a movie, or listening to music. Reassure them it's okay to feel whatever they are feeling—they don't have to put on a cheerful front if they are having a hard time.

If you are not in your Ailey Cat's inner circle, you could still send a card on holidays or their birthday that says something like, "I just wanted to let you know I'm thinking of you and wishing you well."

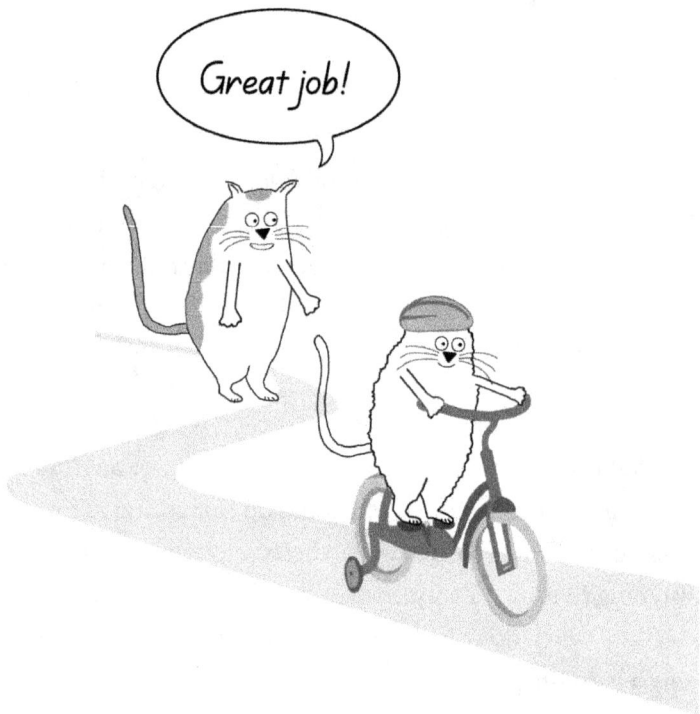

Support Your Ailey Cat's Kittens

If your Ailey Cat has kittens, there may be times when they don't have the capacity to attend to them. It can be very helpful to step up and fill in the gaps, such as giving them rides to school events, taking them shopping, preparing meals with them, doing fun activities together, teaching them essential skills, and so on. It can also be helpful to involve the kittens in celebrations, such as taking them to buy gifts for their Ailey Cat's birthday.

Work with your Ailey Cat and take cues from them about how you can best support their kittens.

Being Sensitive to Your Ailey Cat

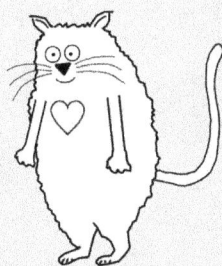

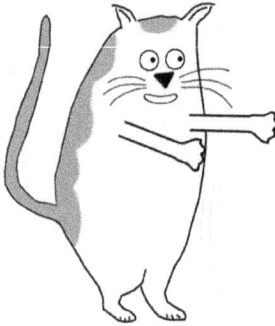

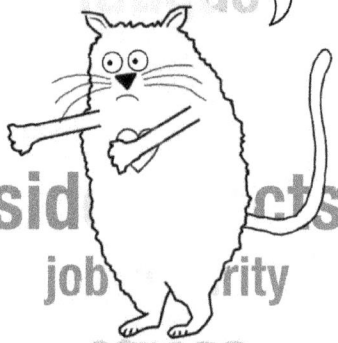

Practice Empathy
with Your Ailey Cat

Simply put, *empathy* is being sensitively aware and in tune with another's feelings. When we are paying attention and notice when our Ailey Cat is having a hard time, it can be a great comfort to step in with some extra tender loving care. The more we understand our Ailey Cats, the better we will be able to intuit how they are feeling, and the better we'll be able to help them.

Empathy can be learned and cultivated. It is a profound practice, but here are some simple suggestions:

- Be curious about your Ailey Cat. Sensitively inquire about their life. For example, ask, "What was it like when you were sick as a kid?" Think about how their life experiences shaped who they are.

- Imagine how you would feel in your Ailey Cat's shoes. How would you want to be treated?

- Inspect your biases and judgments. Release them by reflecting on the idea that no matter what it looks like, everyone is doing the best they can, in any moment.

- Don't assume to know how your Ailey Cat is feeling. Debrief with them after doctor appointments or other happenings by asking, "How was that for you?" or "How did you feel when _____?"

- Explore meditation, in particular *loving-kindness meditation*, in which you learn to cultivate compassion for yourself and others.

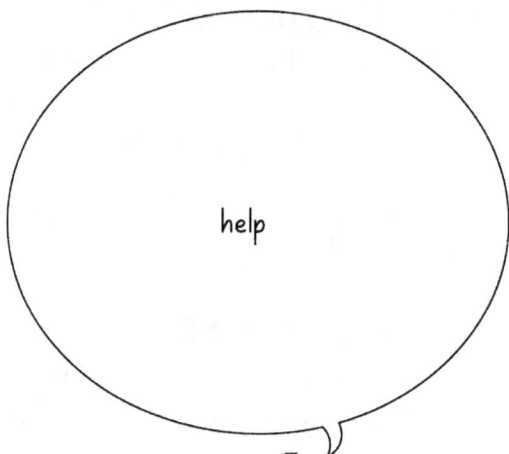

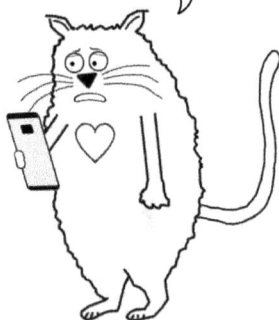

Follow Through
on Commitments

If you have ever had someone cancel on you last minute, you know the sting of being let down. Asking for help can be really hard because, as a culture, we tend to value being independent and self-sufficient. Asking for help can bring up difficult feelings of unworthiness, weakness, or neediness, or fear of being seen as a burden.

It can be particularly disheartening for an Ailey Cat to ask for help in a moment of real need, only to be casually told no, or to not get any response, or to have the person cancel at the last minute, especially if it's regarding something as important as a ride to a medical appointment.

This is why it's really important to:

- Be real about what you can actually commit to (double-check your calendar!).

- Respond to your Ailey Cat's request for help as soon as possible.

- Follow through on any commitments made.

- Stay in communication with your Ailey Cat (for example, let them know a few days before, and then again the day before, that you're still on).

- Give your Ailey Cat as much lead time as possible if you can't follow through (and offer to help make an alternate plan).

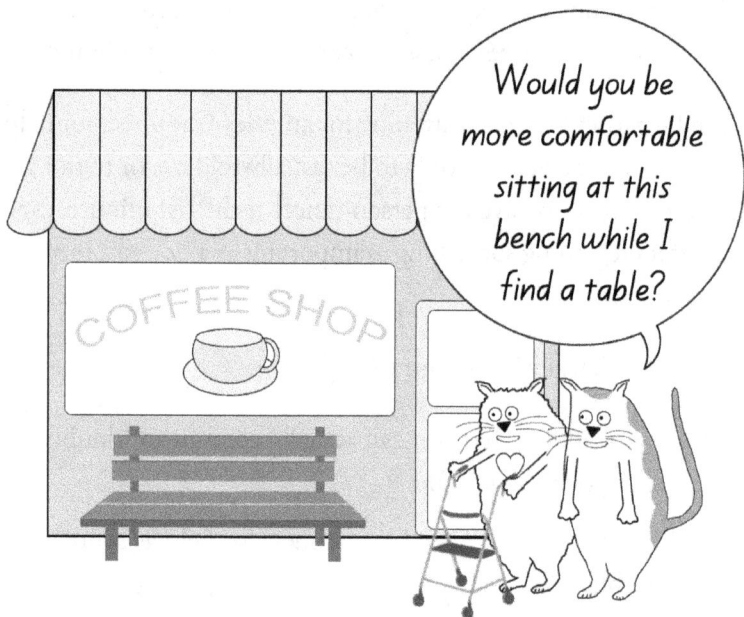

Consider Your Ailey
Cat's Physical Comfort

When you're with your Ailey Cat, pay attention to their comfort and adapt accordingly. You can check in with your Ailey Cat about what they need, but here are some examples of things to pay attention to:

- Situate yourself so your Ailey Cat doesn't need to turn their head or otherwise strain to see you.

- If your Ailey Cat has a hard time standing, make sure they can sit down.

- Speak at a volume that is comfortable to them. Some Ailey Cats may be hard of hearing and find it stressful to struggle to hear someone who is speaking too softly. Some Ailey Cats have sensitive nervous systems and may find it stressful to listen to loud voices or excessive talking.

- Don't require your Ailey Cat to talk if they are too tired. Instead, offer to read to them or just sit quietly and hold space with them. Hold their hand, if they are okay with that.

- Watch for signs that your Ailey Cat is getting tired and it's time for you to leave.

- If you're talking to your Ailey Cat on the phone, don't make them talk longer than they have the energy for.

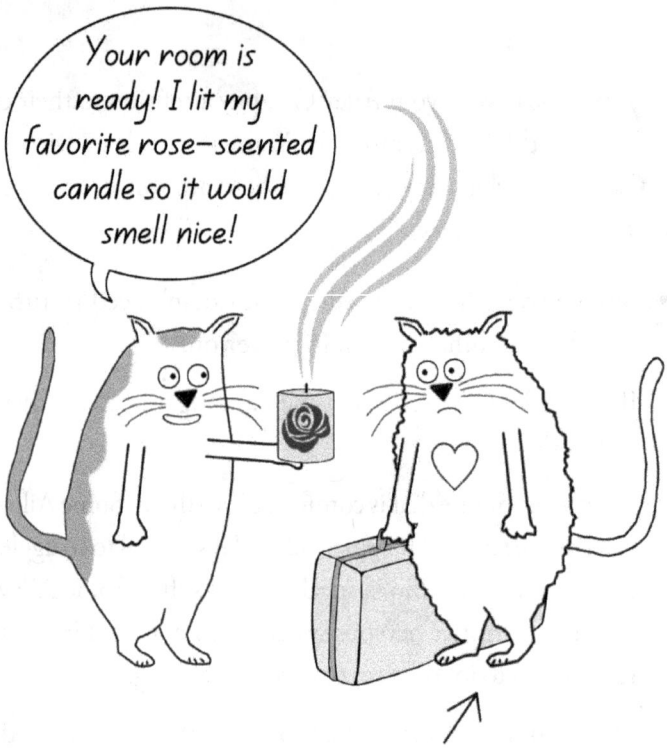

Nausea is a side effect of their
medication. Strong scents can
make it worse.

Consider Your Ailey
Cat's Traveling Needs

When you are hosting your Ailey Cat in your home or traveling with them, think through their condition and what their specific needs are. For example, an Ailey Cat with:

- Arthritis or body pain may need a comfortable mattress

- Respiratory issues or nausea may need a space free of strong odors, fumes, or mold/mildew

- Gastrointestinal (GI) issues may need frequent access to a bathroom

- Mobility challenges may need an accessible space such as a ramp instead of stairs, or a bathroom on the ground level

- Pain or exhaustion (particularly after an intense or invasive medical procedure) may need a quiet, undisturbed space

- A chronic condition may need a special diet

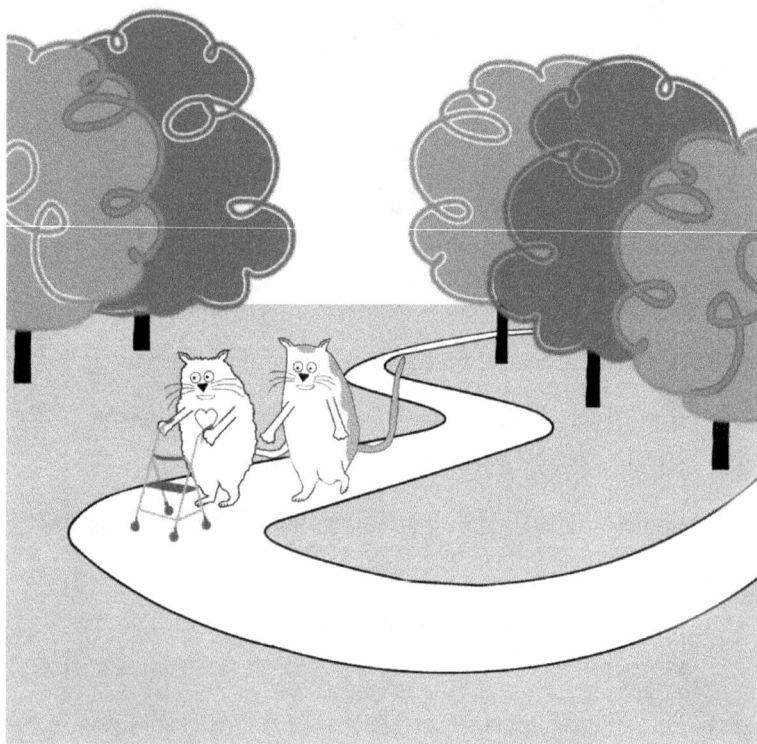

Plan Excursions That Will Be Easy for Your Ailey Cat

I t can be a great gift to help your Ailey Cat get out of the house for a change of scenery. Anticipating things that may be challenging for your Ailey Cat can go a long way toward making things go smoothly. For example:

- If going for a walk, think about the type of terrain—if they have difficulty walking or they use a walker, choose a place with a smooth, paved walkway and give them the option to turn around whenever they get tired.

- If going to a busy, crowded, or noisy place, give them an out if the environment ever becomes too overwhelming for them.

- If going to a restaurant, make sure the building is accessible (for example, it has alternatives to stairs, the entryway is wide enough). Be flexible in choosing a place that works for their specific dietary needs.

Talk through the excursion with your Ailey Cat ahead of time to make sure you know what kind of assistance they need (and whether you can provide it), such as getting in or out of a car, use of a wheelchair, access to a restroom, or door-to-door drop-off. Reassure your Ailey Cat that if they run out of steam at any point, they can request to leave and it won't be a problem.

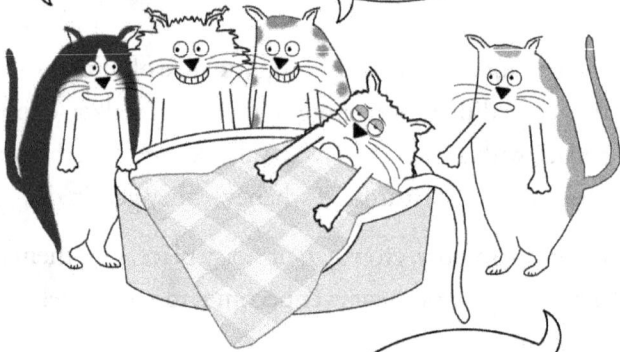

Protect Your Ailey Cat's Space

S ome Ailey Cats may be very sensitive to what's going on around them. Things like noises, people talking, bright lights, and strong smells, for example, can be disturbing. Do what you can to help create and maintain a peaceful space for your Ailey Cat by:

- Conducting yourself so your presence causes the least stress and disturbance possible. Keep your voice low and calm (but loud enough if your Ailey Cat is hard of hearing). Don't wear perfume or other strong scents.

- Creating an environment that reflects your Ailey Cat's preferences (for example, get them sheets and bedding with fabrics they like, ask whether they prefer the blinds open or closed).

- Keeping their space clean and free of clutter. Be mindful about rearranging or moving things—they may have been placed there intentionally, for reasons that are not obvious to you.

- Taking on responsibility for crowd control by monitoring how many people enter the Ailey Cat's room at a time. Intervene if you notice your Ailey Cat being disturbed by someone or something (recognizing that it may not always be possible to intervene in every situation).

- Posting notes for visitors, such as "Please remove your shoes" or "Try to keep your voices down when Ailey Cat is sleeping."

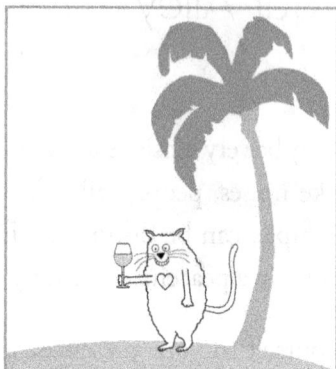

Ailey Cat
Enjoyed a wonderful vacation!

Binx
Wow, you must be feeling better! I thought the chemo would've knocked you out—sounds like your treatments are going well? Didn't you also have a PET scan recently?

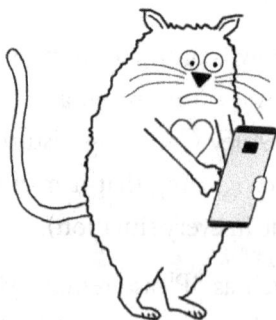

Upset that personal medical details were shared in a comment on social media.

Respect Your Ailey Cat's Privacy, Especially on Social Media

I t should go without saying that information about your Ailey Cat's health condition should remain confidential, but given the nature of social media it bears repeating. Keep in mind that what's happening with your Ailey Cat is *their* story and it is up to them what they want to share and what they want to keep private.

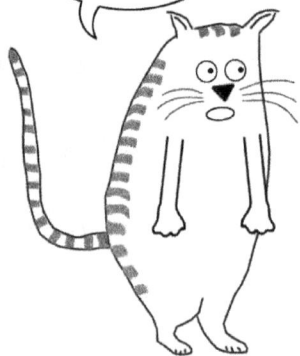

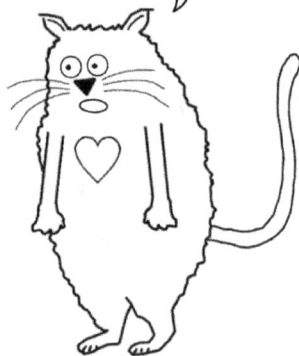

Be Sensitive About Your
Ailey Cat's Prognosis

Having a serious or chronic health condition may lead your Ailey Cat to consider their mortality. Depending on their condition and prognosis, or trajectory of decline, an Ailey Cat may be faced with how much time they may have left and how they want to spend that time. It's an intensely personal consideration and one that is due the utmost sensitivity and respect.

If you are the primary Care Cat, you will need to know the prognosis to better understand what to expect in terms of needs and care. Sometimes your Ailey Cat won't want to know this information, and that's their prerogative.

If you are not the primary Care Cat but still in a supporting role:

- Don't ask your Ailey Cat what their prognosis is.

- Don't ask what the prognosis is for others with the same condition.

- Don't offer a prognosis based on research you've done.

- Don't gossip with others about how much time you think your Ailey Cat has left.

- Don't comment on how others with the same illness have fared.

- Allow your Ailey Cat's healing journey to be a mystery.

- If your Ailey Cat does want to talk about their prognosis, listen with sensitivity (see the tip *"Listen, Be Present, Be a Witness"*).

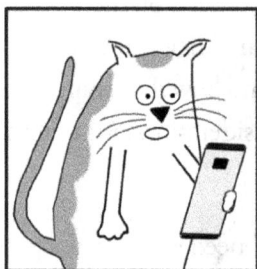

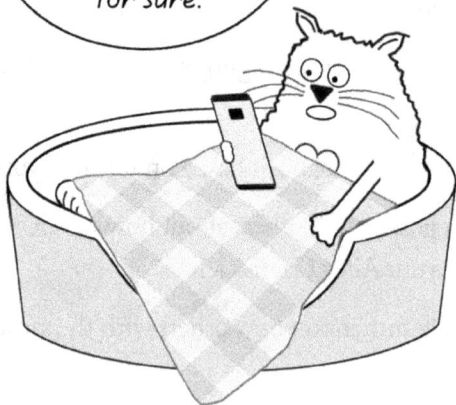

Respect That Your Ailey Cat May Be Immunocompromised

A iley Cats who are dealing with a serious or chronic health condition may have a *compromised immune system*. This means that if they are exposed to other illnesses, they can have a harder time fending them off. Always err on the side of caution when it comes to potentially exposing your Ailey Cat to other illnesses. Let them know in advance if you are having symptoms—never surprise your Ailey Cat by showing up to help and announcing you're sick.

Ask your Ailey Cat ahead of time what they need in order to feel safe and protected. If you have a cold or sore throat, or any other ailment, it's better not to visit your Ailey Cat until you are well.

When you do visit, wash your hands as soon as you walk into their home and ask if they would like you to wear a mask.

Talking With
Your Ailey Cat

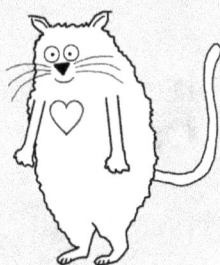

deep listening

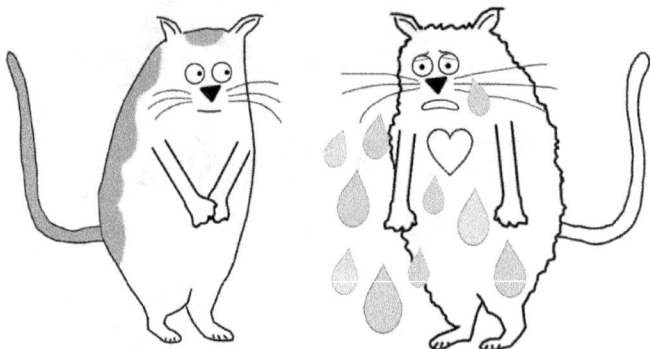

**fully present
with
Ailey Cat**

paying attention

allowing silence

being a witness

being nonreactive

feeling kindness
and compassion

Listen, Be Present,
Be a Witness

One of the greatest gifts you can give your Ailey Cat is to just listen—without giving advice, without trying to fix anything, without trying to cheer them up. Hold space for them, which means being quiet, stopping talking, and listening deeply, giving your Ailey Cat your full attention and presence. This can be challenging because we're not used to silence and often fill it with nervous talking or giving advice.

If your Ailey Cat needs to process their experiences, give them the floor and let them talk or cry or vent or even laugh—whatever comes up for them. *Don't try to talk your Ailey Cat out of their feelings* (for example, avoid saying, "Don't say that—you're going to be fine!"). If your Ailey Cat apologizes for being overly emotional, you could say, "It's okay, I can handle it."

If you find this difficult, practice tuning into your breath and feeling your feet on the floor. Think of your role as bearing witness. You don't need to say anything, except perhaps a very occasional "I'm sorry" or even just "Yeah" to affirm their feelings. Allowing longer periods of silence gives your Ailey Cat space to really feel into their experience and gather their thoughts before they begin speaking again.

Offering your time, presence, and attention based on connection and love, without trying to fix a problem, is powerful medicine.

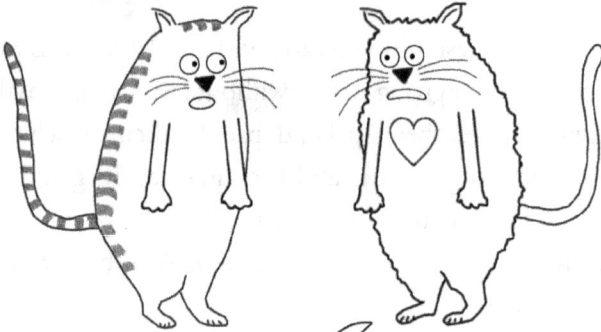

Consider Alternatives to Asking "How Are You?"

We often ask others, "How are you?" without giving it much thought. That can be a loaded question for Ailey Cats.

Instead, ask "How are you *today*?" This shows that you recognize that they have good days and bad days (or moments), and that you are showing genuine care in the present moment.

Depending on the situation and your relationship to the Ailey Cat, you could also say:

- "I've been thinking about you."
- "It's nice to see you."

When you leave a voicemail message or send a text to your Ailey Cat, instead of asking "How are you?" which puts the onus on your Ailey Cat to respond, you could say:

- "I'm thinking of you."
- "Hoping all is going well."
- "Wishing you the best."

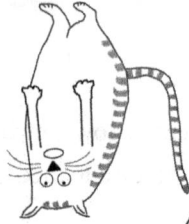

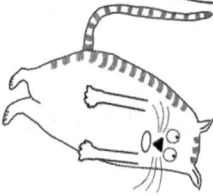

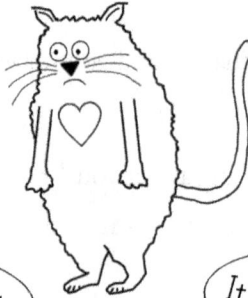

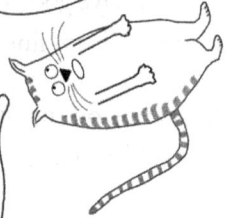

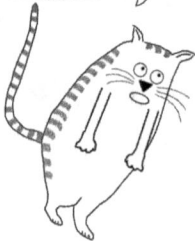

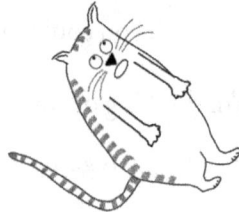

Avoid Platitudes

People often attempt to comfort an Ailey Cat by offering platitudes. Platitudes are rarely helpful because instead of making an Ailey Cat feel better, they stop them from expressing real feelings.

If you don't know what to say to your Ailey Cat, that's okay. You don't have to comfort them. You don't have to fix their distress. You don't have to say anything profound. It's better to say something honest and from the heart, such as:

- "I don't know what to say, but I'm sad for you."
- "I've been thinking about you and hoping you're okay even though I know you're not okay."
- "I don't know what to say, I'm just so sorry."
- "It's not fair, you don't deserve this."

Even if what you say comes out awkwardly, most Ailey Cats will appreciate that you're trying your best.

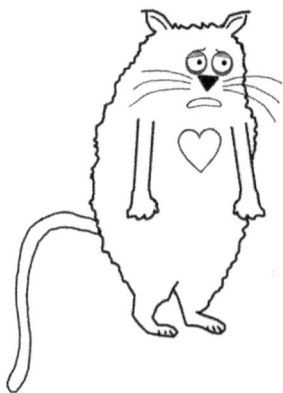

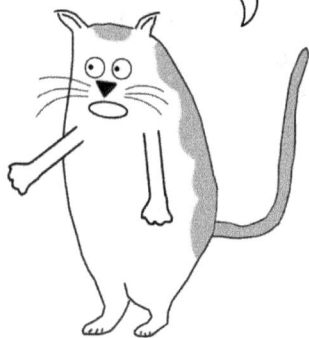

Avoid Toxic Positivity

Toxic positivity is a belief that everyone should maintain a positive attitude even when they are going through a really difficult time. Like platitudes, toxic positivity is not helpful. It doesn't leave space for your Ailey Cat to express their full range of feelings and tends to shut down communication.

So, avoid saying anything to your Ailey Cat that begins with either "Look on the bright side…" or "At least…" Instead, just bear witness to how they are feeling. You may not even need to say anything in response; perhaps it was helpful enough for your Ailey Cat to tell someone how bad they feel.

If it feels appropriate to say something in response, you could say something that validates their feelings and experience, such as:

- "I hear you, it's terrible."

- "You're going through a really difficult passage and doing the best you can; remember to be gentle with yourself."

- "It seems like you're having a totally natural response to awful circumstances. I'm sorry you have to deal with this."

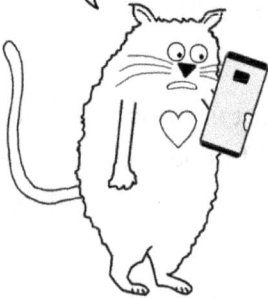

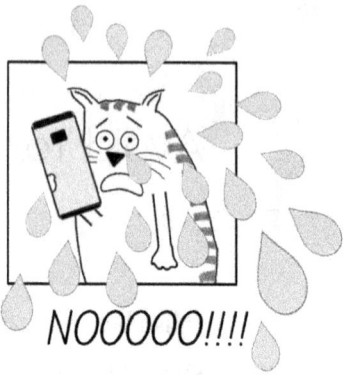

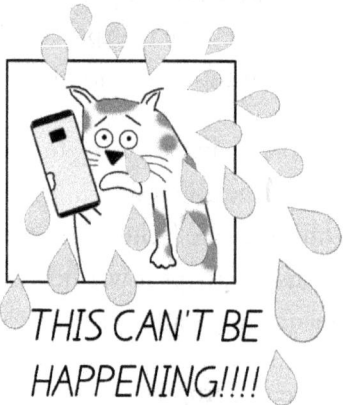

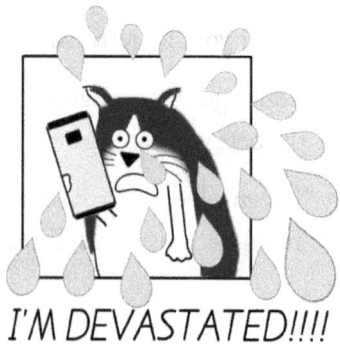

Don't Make Your
Ailey Cat Comfort You

Ailey Cats are not the only ones affected by their illness—it affects all the people in their life. Ailey Cats appreciate that they matter to others and that others may also be experiencing intense emotions regarding their illness. Just be aware that your Ailey Cat may not have the bandwidth to handle anyone else's strong emotions or to provide comfort.

There are times when an Ailey Cat may need to share difficult news, such as adverse test results. Having to deal with the intense emotional reactions of others, even though it's an expression of how much the other person cares, can take energy the Ailey Cat doesn't have.

There may be times when it's helpful to your Ailey Cat to have a good cry along with you. There may be other times when it's better to process your emotions with your own support people.

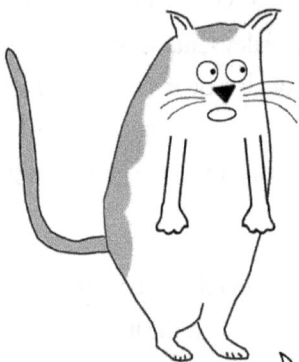

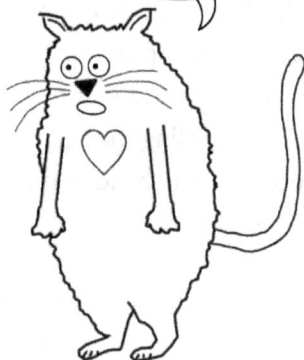

Don't Worry If You Say or Do the "Wrong" Thing

Providing sensitive care is a skill that improves with time and practice. As we're learning, there will be times when we mess up and say or do something insensitive. And that's okay! In those instances, instead of getting defensive or collapsing in shame, go easy on yourself and acknowledge it, responding with something like:

- "I'm sorry, that was insensitive of me. I wasn't thinking."

- "I messed up and said/did the wrong thing. This is new territory to me. I'll be more sensitive in the future."

- "You're absolutely right. I didn't mean to hurt you. I'm sorry, I'll do better."

Most Ailey Cats will appreciate that you mean well and are trying your best in a new situation.

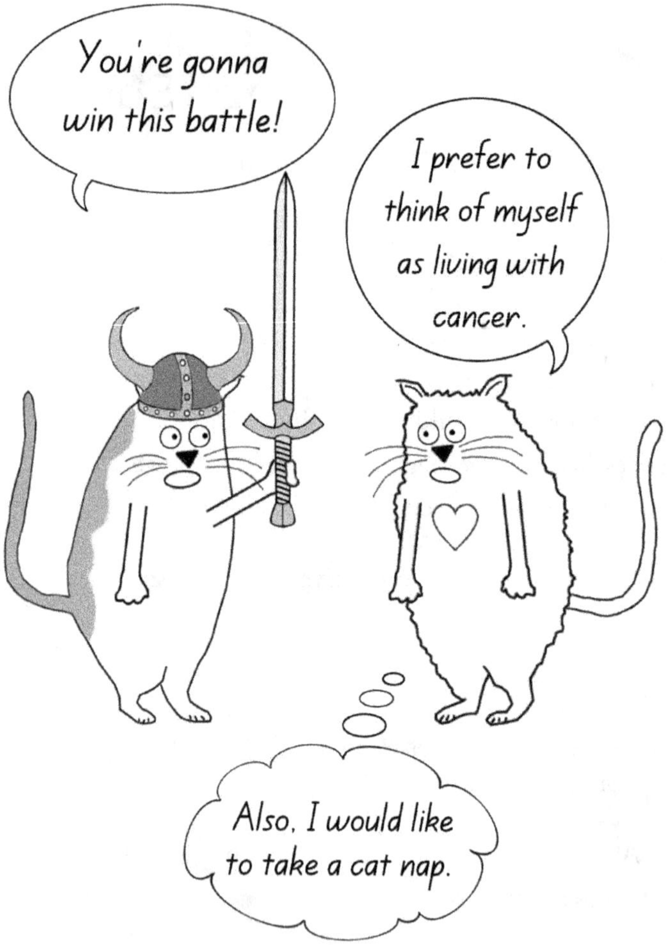
You're gonna win this battle!
I prefer to think of myself as living with cancer.
Also, I would like to take a cat nap.

Avoid Framing Their Healing Journey as a Battle

A lot of the language around dealing with a serious illness or chronic health condition is framed in terms of fighting a battle. This may not resonate with every Ailey Cat, as it implies losers and winners. In other words, if an Ailey Cat doesn't recover, they have somehow lost or failed.

It's helpful to keep in mind that what "winning," "healed," and "healthy" mean in the context of dealing with a serious or chronic illness is different for each Ailey Cat. "Success" is subjective when dealing with so many challenges.

Take a cue from your Ailey Cat on how they talk about their healing journey. You can also check in with your Ailey Cat and ask, "Does it bother you when I talk about this like winning a battle?" If your Ailey Cat can't relate to that metaphor, you could instead express encouragement by saying things like, "I'm here for you," or "I'll do everything I can to help you get through this."

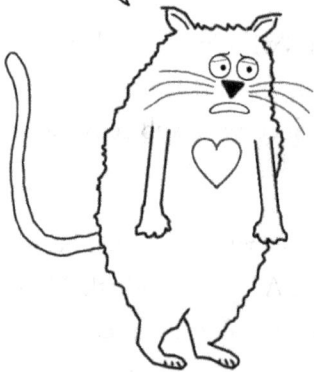

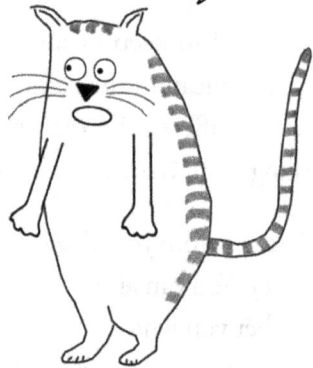

Be Mindful When Making Illness Comparisons

People have a natural impulse to want to relate to what someone else is going through. Oftentimes this is shared by offering similar experiences from their own life. But it's important to appreciate that, unless you've experienced the same illness at the same severity as your Ailey Cat, it may be better to refrain from offering comparisons.

It's not that you can never offer your own life experiences; rather, it's *how* you frame it. Try to present your story in a way that doesn't diminish your Ailey Cat's experience. You might preface your comparison with: "I know it's not the same as what you're going through, but when I was in the hospital for _____ I felt _____."

Additionally, be mindful when complaining about minor health issues to your Ailey Cat. It can be challenging for them to be sympathetic when someone complains about a minor ailment after they've endured an intense or painful medical procedure.

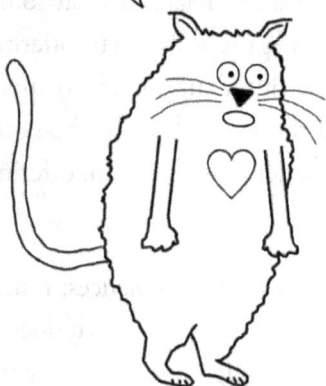

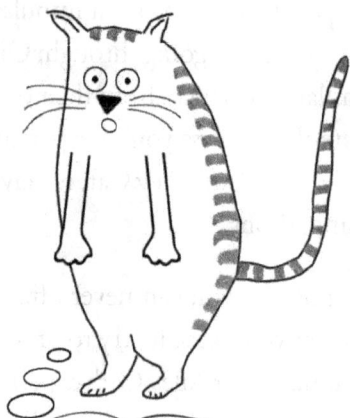

Say the Name of the Illness Aloud

This is mostly about the "C word": cancer. People are often afraid to say it out loud, concerned that it may upset the Ailey Cat or make others uncomfortable. It can feel strange to an Ailey Cat to have their life completely upended by cancer and at the same time have it feel taboo to actually say "cancer" out loud. This can also get in the way of having real conversations about the reality of life with cancer and cancer treatments.

You could check in with your Ailey Cat and say, "I'm noticing how uncomfortable it feels to me to say the word 'cancer' out loud. How does it make you feel? Would you prefer it if I said it?" Take your cue from your Ailey Cat.

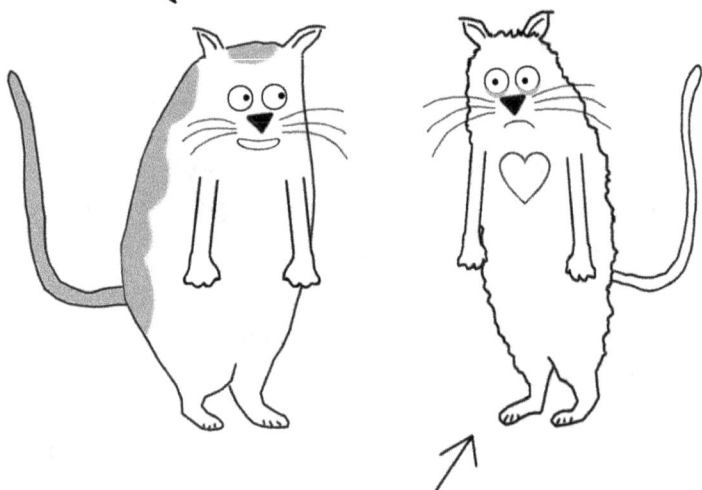

Don't Make a Big Deal of Your Ailey Cat's Appearance

Your Ailey Cat's physical appearance could change over time for a variety of reasons, such as the progression of their illness, certain medical procedures, medication side effects, stress, or anxiety. If you haven't seen them in a while and you are surprised by their appearance, take it in stride and don't make a big deal of it. Instead, just say, "I'm happy to see you." If your Ailey Cat has lost weight, don't compliment them on it since the weight loss came at such a high price.

Relating to
Your Ailey Cat

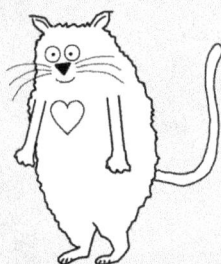

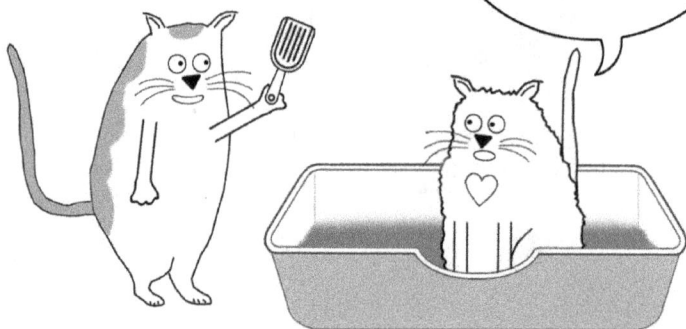

Understand That Dignity is an Important Part of Caregiving

Your Ailey Cat may need help with physical tasks such as bathing or showering, getting in and out of bed or a wheelchair, or eating. It can be embarrassing to need help with tasks that previously were extremely private, such as using the toilet. So, keep in mind that it's not just the doing of these tasks, but *how* you do them, that's important.

Try to preserve your Ailey Cat's dignity as much as possible. Depending on the task and how much your Ailey Cat is able to do for themself, it could mean maximizing privacy by looking away while they're getting dressed, maintaining as much personal space as possible, or giving them a towel to drape over their lap while using the toilet. If your Ailey Cat needs help changing soiled clothing, communicate that it's nothing to be ashamed of by being nonreactive, calm, and reassuring, perhaps by saying, "This happens to a lot of people, I'll take care of this, no problem."

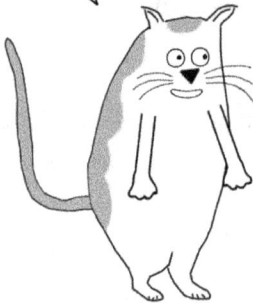

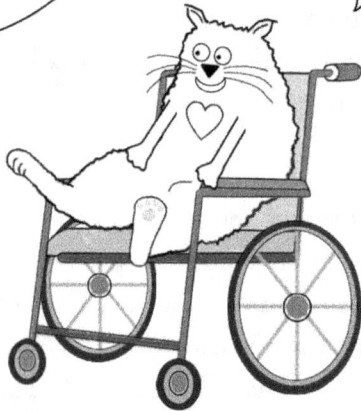

Encourage Normalcy

A void defining your Ailey Cat by their illness, even when their illness is the focus of much of your attention. Encourage normalcy by talking about ordinary things.

Even if your Ailey Cat's attention is, by necessity, focused on managing their health condition, it can be a welcome relief for them to talk about something else: the weather, current events, hobbies, memories, whatever. Check in with your Ailey Cat and see what they'd prefer.

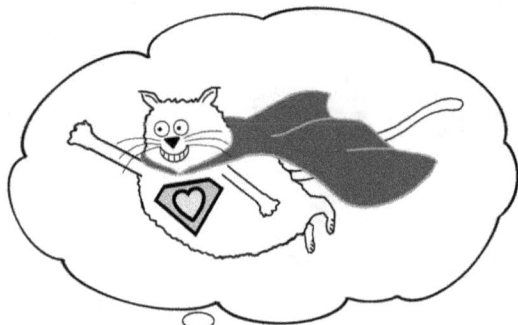

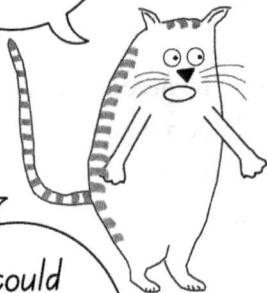

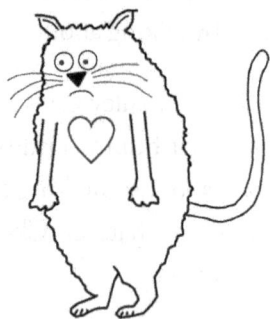

Recognize That Your Ailey Cat is an Ordinary Person Going Through an Extraordinary Experience

Some people express profound admiration for an Ailey Cat's ability to keep going, almost as if it were the result of superhuman strength. This can actually come across as insincere (or a projection of the person's own fears), because Ailey Cats don't have any more strength than anyone else; their strength is just being tested in a way that others may not have experienced.

What's intended to be praise can instead feel alienating, as it reinforces the illusion that being healthy, independent, and productive is the norm, and that if something outside this norm strikes someone, they become a sort of tragic figure who is either pitied or sanctified, instead of just being treated like an ordinary person dealing with life.

That said, some Ailey Cats do find it encouraging when someone sincerely tells them, "You are very strong." It's okay to test the waters and see how your Ailey Cat responds, or just ask them, "Does it bother you when I say that?"

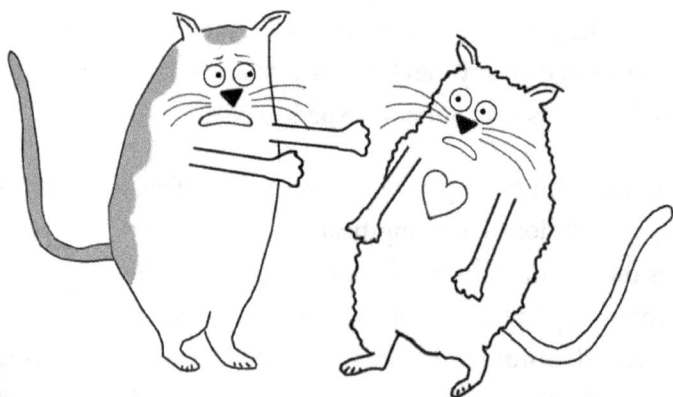

Treat Your Ailey Cat as an Empowered Person, Not a Victim

There is a difference between supporting an Ailey Cat and feeling sorry for them. The difference is that support is *empowering*; pitying is *disempowering*. Pitying can imply that your Ailey Cat is at the mercy of their health condition; that they are weak, childlike, or broken; or that there is something fundamentally "wrong" with them. This can be off-putting to Ailey Cats because, no matter what challenges life throws at them, they are still human beings with sovereignty and agency over their lives.

This is not to say that you can't express sympathy if your Ailey Cat is in pain or otherwise suffering. Hold space for them to tell you how they're feeling or what they're going through, and affirm it, rather than responding with, "Oh, you poor thing!" It's about being sympathetic to the suffering but also respecting the intelligence of the person and their healing process.

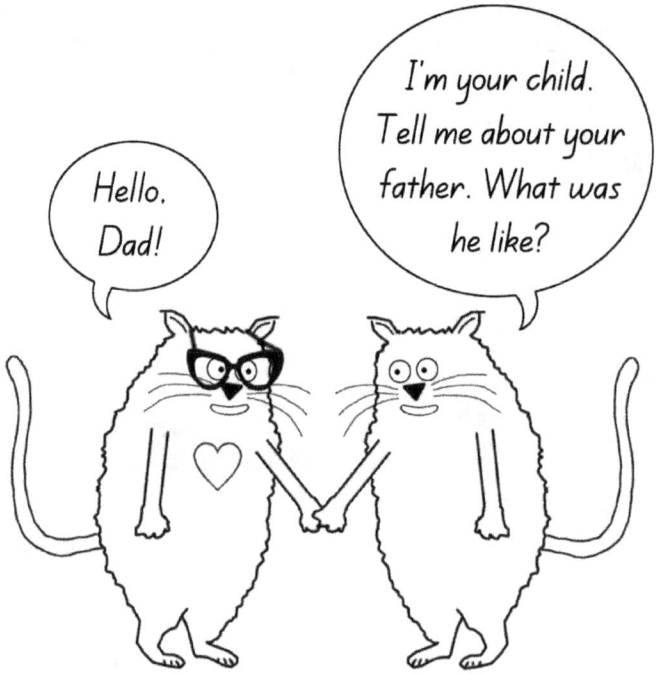

Ailey Cat has dementia from Alzheimer's.

Accept That Your Relationship with Your Ailey Cat Will Change

When you care for a loved one who has a serious illness, the relationship changes. The person you knew as a partner or parent or friend may not be able to show up in that role any longer. With some illnesses, your Ailey Cat may not even recognize you.

While this passage has the potential to deepen your relationship in unexpected ways as you go to this new and profound place together, it can be really challenging and, at times, heartbreaking. For example, it can be intense to help a parent bathe and see them naked or to change their soiled clothing. Interestingly, it can also be very poignant to meet a loved one in their vulnerability, or to care for a parent as they cared for you when you were a child.

These changing relationship dynamics can also come with a lot of grief as you let go of the way things used to be. It can be helpful to seek out grief resources such as books, websites, and support groups.

Setting Aside What You Think You Know

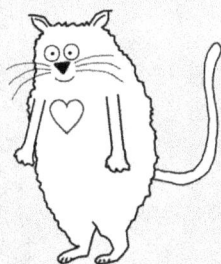

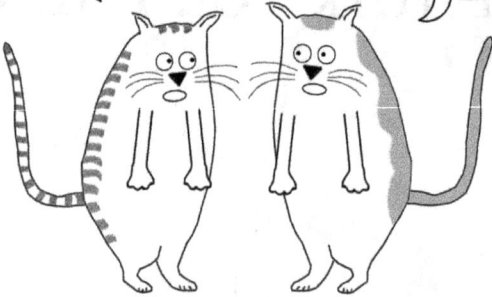

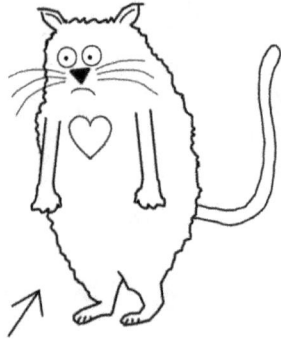

Inspect Your Biases
and Judgments

A iley Cats often receive a lot of judgment couched as advice, such as, "You would feel better if you ate healthier food, exercised more, and got enough sleep." Or they get insinuations that they are exaggerating their condition to get attention or to avoid work.

Ailey Cats know when they are being judged, and it hurts. It's also very likely that no one is harder on Ailey Cats than they already are on themselves. Judgment doesn't serve any good purpose and it inhibits kindness and compassion.

If you notice you have biases or are judgmental toward your Ailey Cat, it can be helpful to:

- Acknowledge that we all have compensatory strategies for comfort (no one wants to be judged for eating chocolate!).

- Think about your beliefs and reflect on why they are triggering for you (sometimes what we judge is a reflection of something about ourselves that we haven't dealt with).

- Appreciate that no one *deserves* to suffer, even if you don't agree with their life choices.

- Get to know your Ailey Cat's life story to better understand and hold compassion for their reality.

- Practice a loving-kindness meditation in relation to your Ailey Cat.

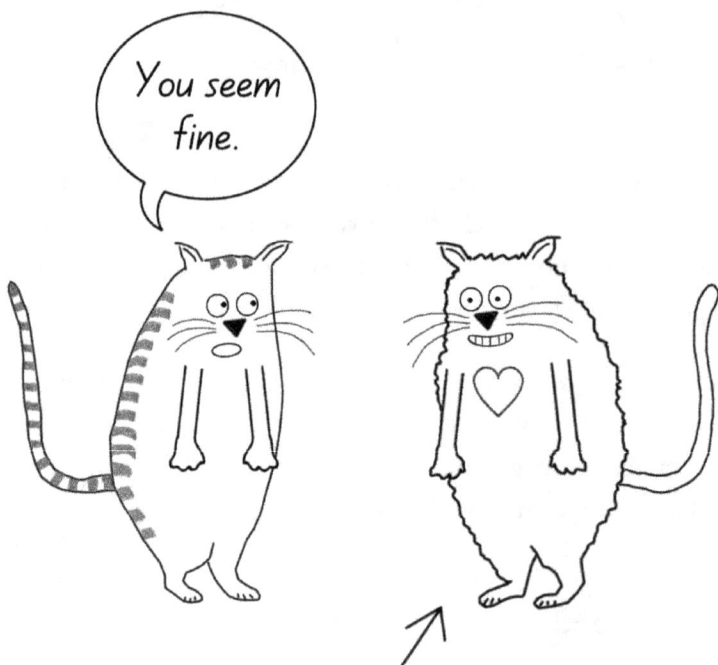

Lives with severe pain and fatigue. Has spent thousands of dollars over the years seeing doctors and specialists, getting tests, and trying many different treatment plans to manage their disease. Pushes themself beyond their limit every day to show up and contribute the best they can.

Understand That
Not All Illness Is Visible

You may not be able to gauge how your Ailey Cat is feeling just by looking for outward signs of illness. This is particularly true for Ailey Cats with chronic conditions such as rheumatoid arthritis, chronic fatigue syndrome, diabetes, celiac disease, lupus, and others.

When they appear to be having a "good" day, some people come to the false conclusion that Ailey Cats must be faking their extremely debilitating or painful symptoms on other days. The reality is that Ailey Cats with chronic conditions don't fake their symptoms; they are more likely to fake being *okay*. Ailey Cats often struggle to appear "well" in order to participate with people or activities in a way that feels ordinary and "normal."

You can help your Ailey Cat by:

- Asking how they are feeling, even if they appear to be "well"

- Believing what they tell you without judgment

- Letting them know that you care how they are feeling

- Reassuring them that you can be flexible and adjust plans to accommodate their needs

- Standing by them over time

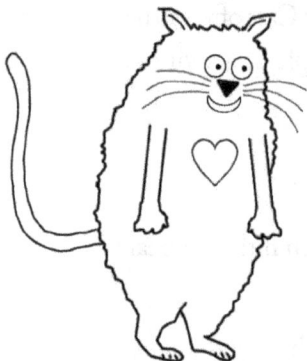

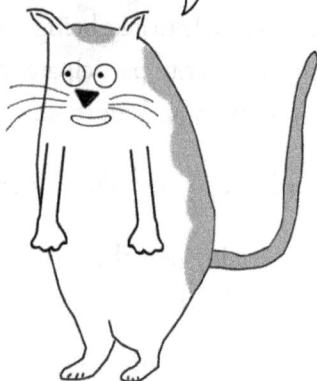

Respect Your Ailey
Cat's Autonomy

Ailey Cats have to make a lot of tough decisions. On top of that, they sometimes have to contend with very strong opinions from well-intentioned family and friends. It's important to respect your Ailey Cat's autonomy, even if you disagree with their choices or believe you know more than they do.

The issue is not always that you are offering an opinion, alternative point of view, or information that you want them to consider—it's *how* you offer it. Instead of saying, "You should _____," first ask your Ailey Cat if they are open to hearing what you think.

- If they say no, let it go.

- If they say yes, ask if they've already heard of or considered your idea. If they haven't, frame your suggestion in a way that doesn't cast aspersions on the choices they've made so far or imply that they have poor judgment. You might say, "I'm wondering what you think of this idea, how it feels to you…"

There may be times when you *are* "right," and it's frustrating when your Ailey Cat doesn't want to hear it. Sometimes, the only thing you can do is plant a seed. Things may need to run their course before they can see the importance of what you were saying, and that is their life lesson. You may have to be okay with the knowledge that you did everything you could.

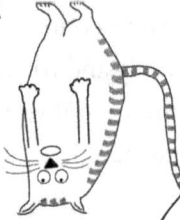

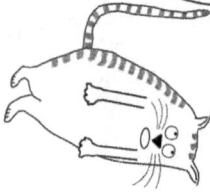

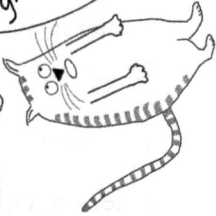

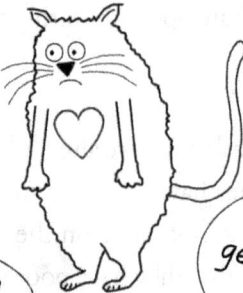

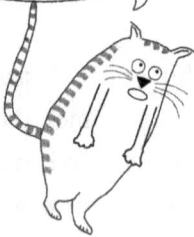

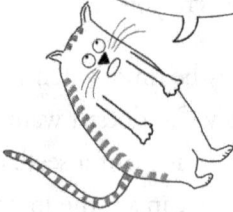

Offer Advice Only
When Requested

People have the best of intentions, but they often confuse *giving advice* with *being helpful*. Giving unsolicited advice is rarely helpful, but it is particularly unhelpful to an Ailey Cat. Their healing journey is not a problem for you to solve. You cannot "fix" them. You cannot cure them.

Your advice may also come off as patronizing, as it's possible (and probably likely) that your Ailey Cat has already considered what you are suggesting (for example, "You should get more exercise").

It can be exhausting for an Ailey Cat to field unsolicited advice from others. Unless your Ailey Cat explicitly asks for your advice, it's best not to offer it.

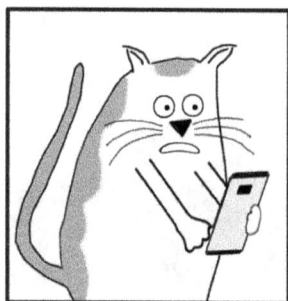

I'm getting on the next plane! I can stay in a hotel or at your place. Let me know what works for you and how long you want me to stay. Is there an airport shuttle?

Feels like they are a friendship fail if they don't show up right away.

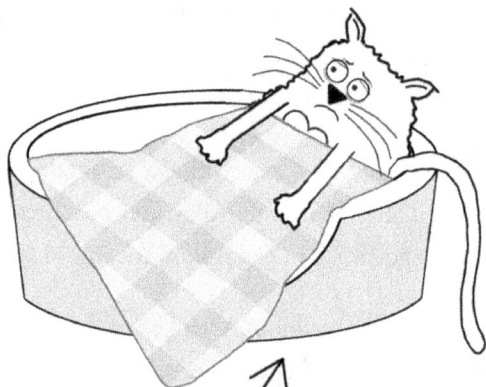

Wants friend to wait (or not come at all) because they don't have the energy to see anyone or respond to questions.

Let Go of What You Think Help Looks Like

You may have a definite idea of what it means to be helpful. However, what your Ailey Cat actually needs might be very different from what *you* think they need.

For example, when a loved one is in crisis, our first impulse is often to rush to their side. We may feel guilty if we don't drop everything and show up for them. This may not be what your Ailey Cat wants or needs, as they may not have the energy to engage with people.

When supporting your Ailey Cat, it's important not to project what *you* would want onto them. Instead, really listen to whatever your Ailey Cat is telling you they need (or don't need).

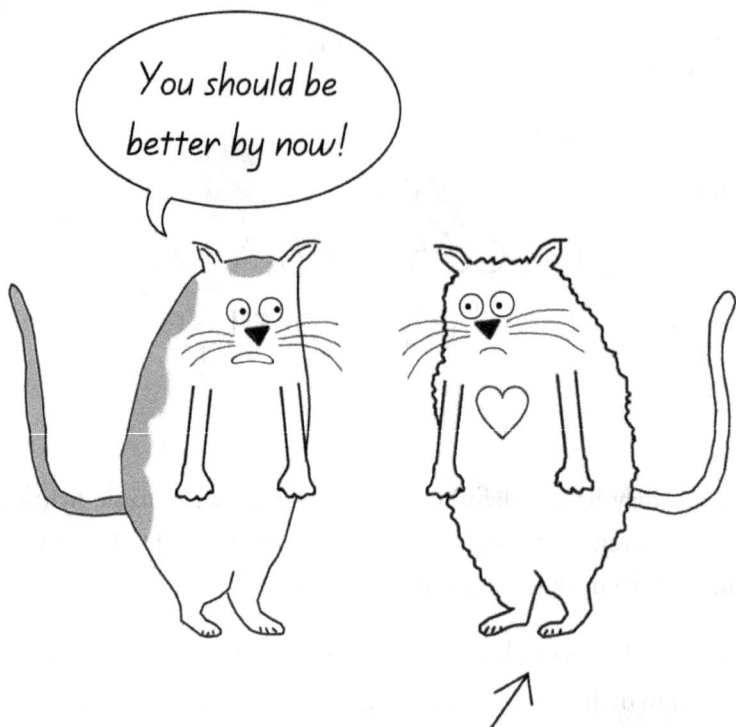

Is living with an incurable systemic
autoimmune disease that requires
long-term medication and care
strategies to maintain a quality of
life that still means coping with
aching, burning body pain, and
extreme exhaustion.

Allow Your Ailey Cat's Health Journey to Have Its Own Timeline

Ailey Cats, especially those with chronic health conditions, must often contend with the misconception that all illness follows a particular course or trajectory, after which they should be recovered. The truth is that illness can be complex and mysterious, and there are illnesses for which there is no known cure. It is sobering to acknowledge that it's possible to become ill and never fully recover.

We can't put a timeline on something we can't understand, and it's impossible to fully know what's going on with someone's body and illness. Ailey Cats typically go to great lengths to manage their health and can experience great frustration themselves at being ill for so long, feeling like they did everything "right" and wondering why they aren't better.

You can help your Ailey Cat by:

- Holding space, without frustration or judgment, for their healing journey to take however long it takes

- Not framing their healing journey in terms of success or failure (insinuating they are failing if they aren't getting better)

- Releasing any preconceived ideas you have about what "healthy" means

Advocating for Your Ailey Cat

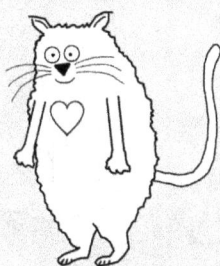

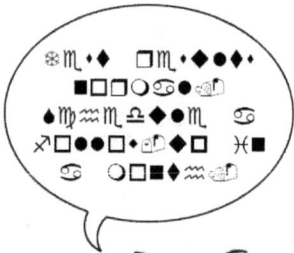

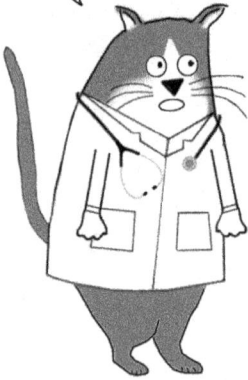

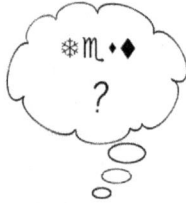

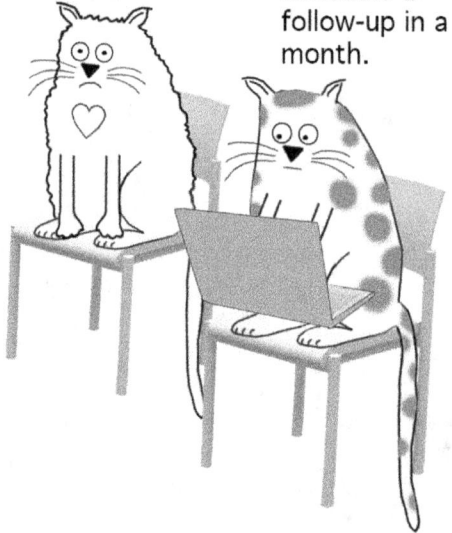

Test results were normal. Schedule a follow-up in a month.

Be an Advocate for Your Ailey Cat in the Health-Care System

For many Ailey Cats, navigating the various systems involved in health care (for example, medical, social services, insurance) can be incredibly stressful and confusing. It can be a great help to an Ailey Cat to have someone who will proactively look out for their best interests and advocate for them. This may include such things as:

- Sorting out with your Ailey Cat the most important information needed from the doctor prior to an appointment

- Accompanying your Ailey Cat to doctor appointments

- Making sure your Ailey Cat is heard

- Asking clarifying questions

- Taking notes or recording the visit

- Calling insurance companies to sort out issues, such as challenging a claim that was denied coverage

Being an advocate requires some boldness, because it can be intimidating to ask a doctor to slow down or explain something in a different way. But it's a really important service that can relieve your Ailey Cat of a significant burden.

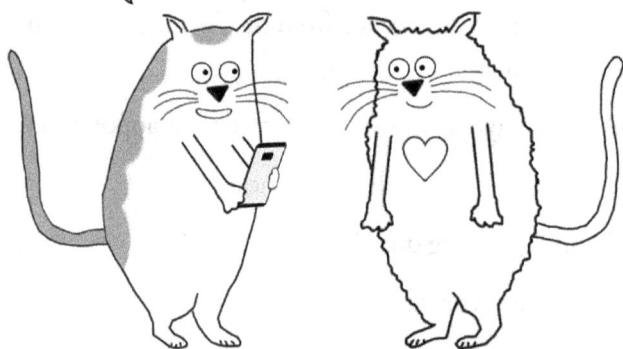

Be an SOS Person or an Emergency Contact

If your Ailey Cat lives alone, they may appreciate having an SOS person who is willing to be available 24/7 if they need help, even if it's in the middle of the night. Knowing that there's someone there gives the Ailey Cat a sense of security. It's important to really commit to this if you offer, because it may turn out that the one night you turn off your phone is the night they need you.

Depending on your Ailey Cat's condition, it may be helpful to support them to get a medical alert bracelet they can use to notify emergency services if they fall or have another type of accident or emergency.

Additionally, some Ailey Cats don't have anyone to list as an emergency contact on their medical forms. Depending on how close you are to the Ailey Cat, you could offer to be that person.

medication side
effects

adverse
reactions

reputable
sources of
medical
information

pharmacy
documentation &
labels

drug
interactions

As requested, I did some
research on side effects.
Here is a summary of what
I think are the most
important things to
consider.

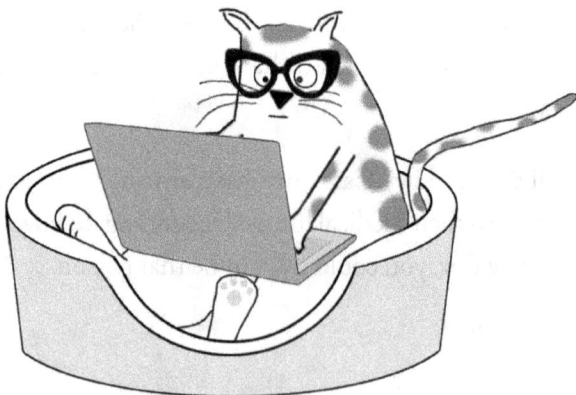

Do Research for Your Ailey Cat

Dealing with a serious or chronic illness can come with a steep learning curve. It takes a lot of time and energy to research the illness itself, learn about treatment options, evaluate medication side effects and drug interactions, figure out how to navigate the medical system, and so many other new things that come with managing a major health issue.

It can be a great relief for an Ailey Cat to hand this task off to someone else. If you take it on, keep in mind that you are offering information for your Ailey Cat to make an informed decision. They may ask what you would recommend, but it's ultimately their decision.

It's also advantageous for Care Cats to research the health condition for their own benefit, because being informed can make you a better support person. But be mindful not to come across as thinking you know more than your Ailey Cat. When talking about what you have learned, you could frame it as: "I was reading about your condition and wanted to see if something I learned matched your experience."

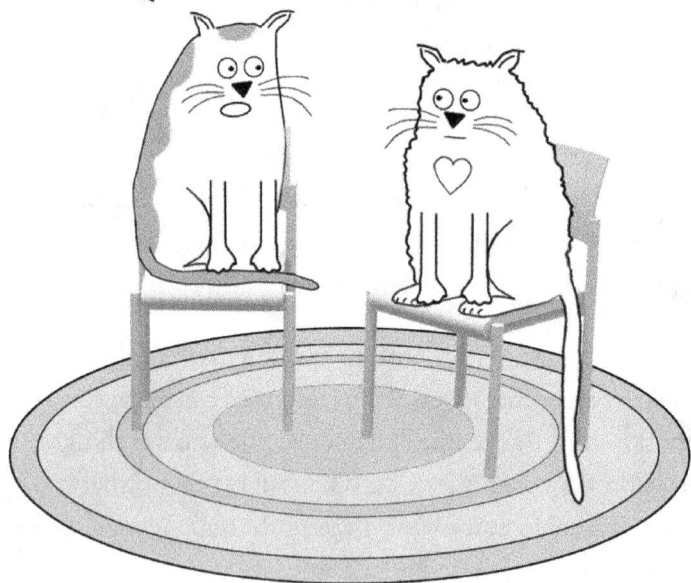

Help Your Ailey Cat Make Decisions

Decision fatigue is something we all experience, but it's even more intense for Ailey Cats. On top of not feeling well, they may be asked to make tough decisions from a selection of choices that all seem terrible.

Your Ailey Cat may greatly appreciate having someone with whom to talk things through, to help arrive at decisions that feel right to them. Keep in mind that your role is to support your Ailey Cat to make a decision and not to insert your opinions about what you think they should do (unless they ask for that).

Asking sensitive, open-ended questions, such as the following, may be useful to help your Ailey Cat get clarity:

- What are the pros and cons of each option?
- What do you see as possible consequences of each option?
- What things are most important to you?
- Is there any additional information you need in order to make a decision?
- Is there anyone else's input you would like before deciding?
- Which sources of information do you trust the most?
- What do you consider a deal-breaker?
- What concerns you the most?
- How does each option feel in your gut?
- If you picture a best- or worst-case scenario, what does that look like?
- What kind of support would you need for each option?

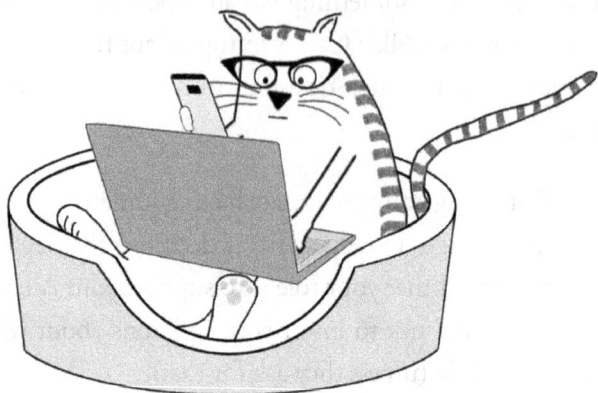

I contacted the insurance company and sorted out the issue with the disputed claim.

Thank you!

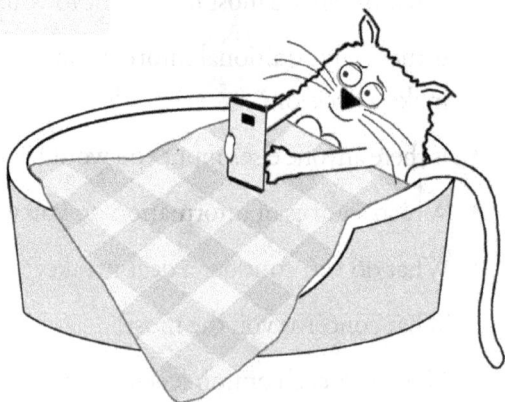

Manage Administrative Tasks

Dealing with a serious or chronic health condition can involve a lot of administrative tasks. Volunteering to take the lead on any of these can be extremely helpful to your Ailey Cat. You could:

- Track doctors' appointments, test dates, results, symptoms, medications, treatments, side effects, insurance bills and payments, and a myriad of other details.

- Coordinate Care Cats and volunteers, scheduling, meals, and more.

- Communicate with doctors, medical centers, and insurance companies, and provide updates to friends and family.

- Manage household tasks, such as opening mail or scheduling bill payments.

Check with your Ailey Cat before taking on any of these tasks, as they require the Ailey Cat to be comfortable trusting others with potentially sensitive and personal information.

Help Your Ailey Cat Complete Advance Directive Forms

I t's really important for everyone (not just Ailey Cats) to have advance directive forms in place so their Care Cats know their preferences. It can be challenging for Ailey Cats to think about these things when they are on a path to recovery, so sensitivity and patience may be required to help them complete this task. Here are some things to consider:

- **Advance Directive** (also known as a living will or Health Care Power of Attorney) is a document that states your medical care wishes if you are unable to. It includes designating a Health Care Proxy to make decisions on your behalf.

- **Financial Power of Attorney** is a legal document in which you authorize someone else to make money decisions for you.

- **POLST (Physician Orders for Life-Sustaining Treatment)** is for people with serious illness; it tells health care providers during a medical emergency what you want.

- **Do Not Resuscitate (DNR)** is completed with your doctor; you select what medical interventions you want if you stop breathing or your heart stops.

- **Organ and Tissue Donation**

- **Executor of a Last Will and Testament** is the person designated in a will drawn up by a lawyer to handle financial affairs after a person has died.

- **5 Wishes** helps someone reflect on their spiritual and emotional values as they imagine the end of life.

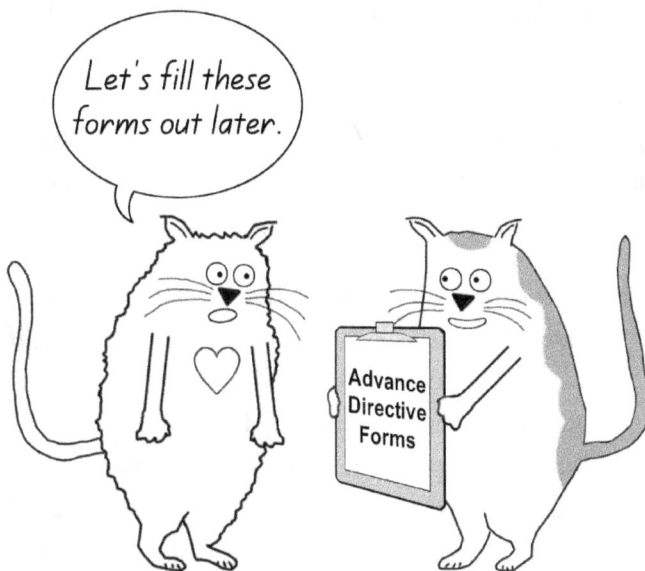

Let's fill these forms out later.

Advance Directive Forms

It would be better to do it now. Completing these forms will help me to know your wishes and feel more confident in my ability to make informed decisions on your behalf if I ever need to. You would be giving me the gift of peace of mind.

Know the Differences Between Hospice, Palliative Care, and Medicare

As a Care Cat, you may find yourself in a position where you need to advocate for additional support for your Ailey Cat. Educating yourself about options sooner rather than later will help you be prepared if or when the time comes. A good place to start is by becoming familiar with *hospice care, palliative care*, and *Medicare*.

- **Hospice care:** Medical care for people who are expected to have six months or less to live. However, qualifying for hospice care doesn't always mean that death is imminent and there's no turning back. Each person and situation is unique. Some people stop hospice care in order to resume curative-based treatments. Some people live longer with hospice care than they would otherwise because the reduction of stress and increase of comfort can benefit health.

- **Palliative care:** This is specialized medical care for people living with a serious illness. It is focused on improving quality of life for patients and caregivers by providing relief from the symptoms and stress of the illness. It's sometimes thought of as "comfort care." People often equate palliative care with end-of-life care, but you don't need to be dying to benefit from palliative care.

- **Medicare and Medicaid:** Medicare is a medical insurance program for people over 65 and younger disabled people and dialysis patients. Medicaid is an assistance program for low-income patients' medical expenses. Medicare and Medicaid cover the cost of hospice.

You'll want to do your own research to find out exactly what each has to offer and what your Ailey Cat qualifies for.

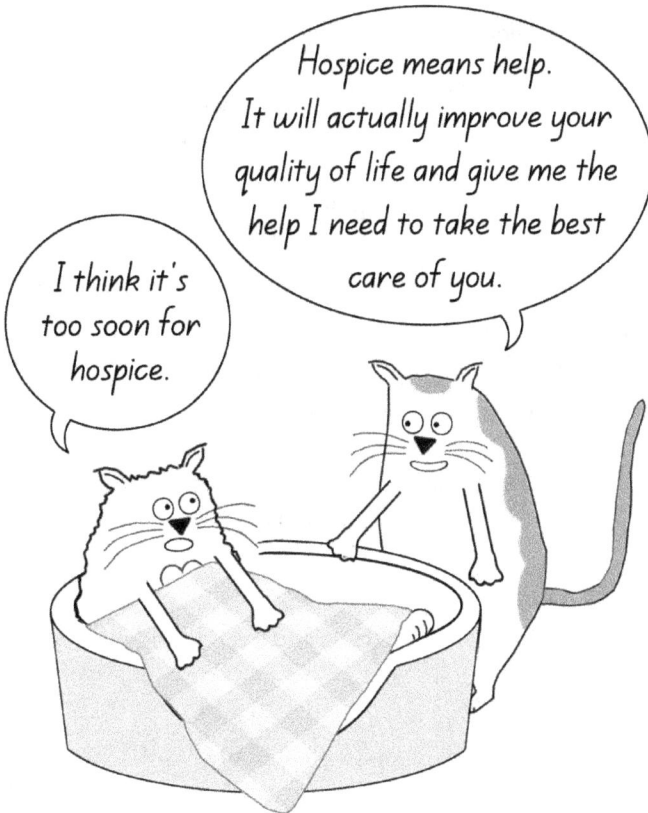

Raise Money for Your Ailey Cat

Living with a serious or chronic health condition is really expensive and can come with the added worry of being unable to work and generate income. It can be a great help to raise money for your Ailey Cat. You can do this in a variety of ways, for example, by:

- Asking people in your inner circle to give money directly to your Ailey Cat

- Creating an online wish list with links where people can purchase items and have them shipped to your Ailey Cat

- Creating an online fundraiser

Online fundraising platforms are often used to help with expenses. They can be easily shared on social media and have the potential to reach a broader audience than just the Ailey Cat's immediate circle. It's also important to consider the downsides:

- It requires the Ailey Cat to disclose their health situation and financial status to the public.

- Ailey Cats are expected to provide regular updates to donors, which takes time and energy, and also vulnerability.

- Someone must act as a "marketer" to circulate the site through social media and make sure it stays current and visible.

- It can be disappointing if a fundraising website isn't successful.

Whatever approach you use, be sure that you and your Ailey Cat have fully considered what's involved, that everyone understands their roles and responsibilities, and it's clear how the money will be given to the Ailey Cat.

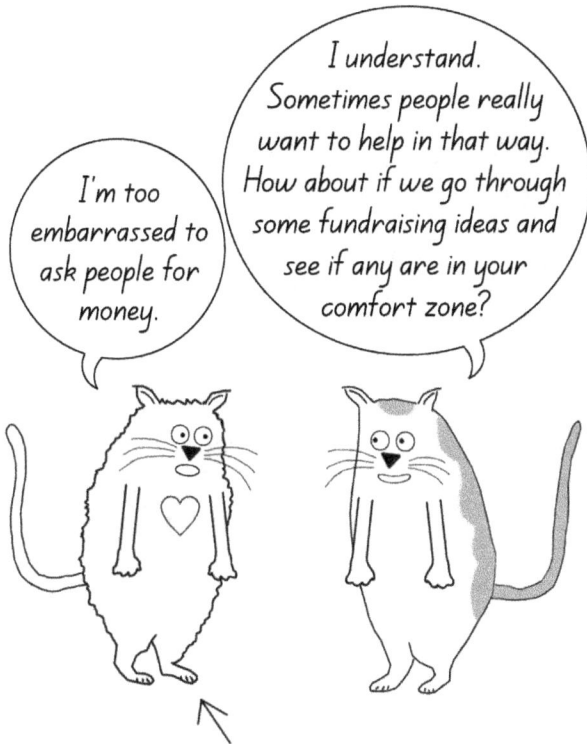

I'm too embarrassed to ask people for money.

I understand. Sometimes people really want to help in that way. How about if we go through some fundraising ideas and see if any are in your comfort zone?

Struggling to cover co-pays for doctor appointments, health insurance premiums, deductibles, tests, home care, food for specialized diet, vitamins and supplements, medical supplies, and more.

Taking Care of Yourself
While Supporting
Your Ailey Cat

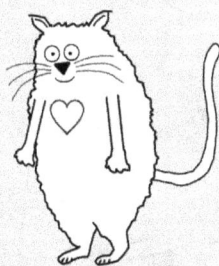

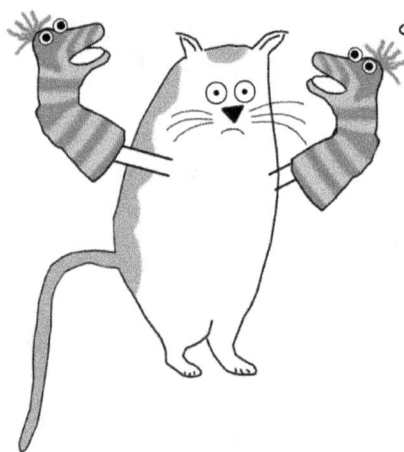

Be Real About What You're Actually Up For

Before offering to help your Ailey Cat, it's important to be clear about what you can realistically offer. Giving out of balance can lead to overwhelm, burnout, or resentment. If you overcommit, you may leave your Ailey Cat in a bind when you can't follow through.

Consider your own boundaries and limits, such as:

- Can you support your Ailey Cat in a balanced, sustainable way?

- Are there others with whom you can form a team to best support your Ailey Cat?

- Can you handle seeing someone you care about in pain, distress, or suffering?

- Are you able to help with Activities of Daily Living (ADLs)? See the next tip, *"Consider Your Comfort Zone for Assisting with Physical Care,"* for details.

- How much time do you realistically have each day or week?

Know that you can set boundaries around what you are willing to give. At the same time, don't discount seemingly small gestures such as sending flowers, cards, gifts, or a thoughtful text. A little can go a long way and make a big difference to your Ailey Cat.

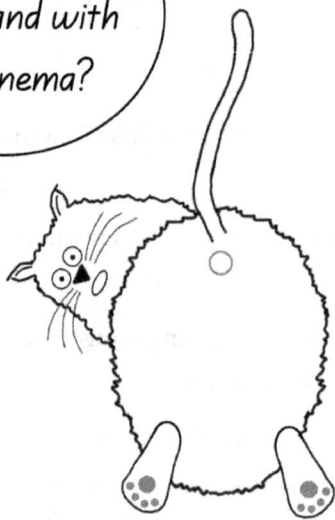

Consider Your Comfort Zone for Assisting with Physical Care

Your Ailey Cat may need help with Activities of Daily Living (ADLs) such as eating, bathing, dressing, toileting, and moving from one place to another. It's important to be clear whether you're up for providing this kind of support. Some tasks require special training, such as moving your Ailey Cat from a lying to a sitting position or from the bed to a wheelchair. You'll need to consider if you're up for that and, if so, find out where you can get the training.

It's natural to feel squeamish about providing personal care, and it's okay if you aren't up to it.

- You could let your Ailey Cat know up front by saying something like, "I'm happy to help with household chores or errands, but I'm just letting you know now that I can't help with any personal care stuff—it makes me too uncomfortable."

- If you're put on the spot, you could say, "I'm sorry, this isn't something I'm comfortable with [or wouldn't be safe for me to do, if it involves heavy lifting], but let's see if we can find someone who is."

Sometimes, there is no one else around to do the task we're uncomfortable doing. Those situations are difficult and sometimes involve setting aside our discomfort and doing the task to the best of our ability.

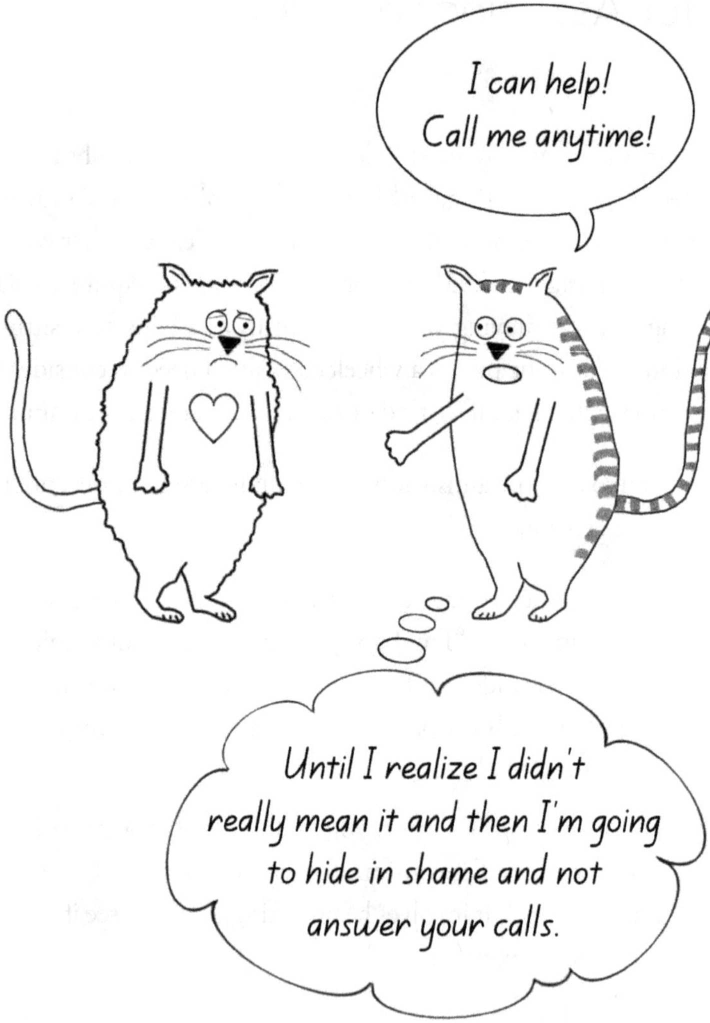
I can help! Call me anytime!
Until I realize I didn't really mean it and then I'm going to hide in shame and not answer your calls.

Allow Yourself to Say No

Saying no to an Ailey Cat who asks for help can be hard. Even though it may sting a bit, most Ailey Cats would rather you be honest and say no than say yes and cancel, or say yes and feel resentful. Here are some ways you could frame a polite decline:

- "I'm sorry, I just can't make it work on Friday, but I could help another day."

- "I'm sorry, I'm just not comfortable doing that task. Is there anything else I could help you with?"

- "I'm glad you reached out and I really want to help, but I'm overwhelmed and not in a place where I can show up for you right now."

- "I'm sorry, I just don't have the bandwidth to help you with this, I wish I could. Would it help if I contacted a couple of other friends to see if they are available?"

- "I really care about you and wish I could be with you 24/7, but I have other obligations."

It's hard when we feel as if we're letting someone down, and the reality is that we can't always stick to our own boundaries. It may feel impossible to say no if your Ailey Cat is in crisis and doesn't have anyone else to ask. This can present an impossible bind—whether to take care of yourself or your Ailey Cat. Unfortunately, our society doesn't provide comprehensive support to those who need a higher level of care, especially for Ailey Cats who live alone and don't have family or community support. So, we do the best we can, in the midst of impossible situations.

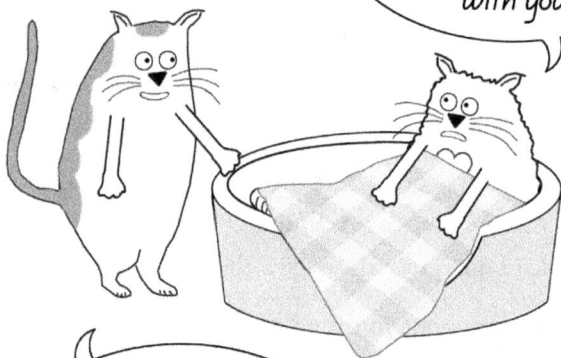

Understand That Caregiving Is a Relationship That Includes You

When it comes to supporting an Ailey Cat who requires a high level of care, people often presume incorrectly that Care Cats have a limitless supply of time, energy, and compassion, or that one cat can do it all.

Misconceptions can also be self-imposed. Some Care Cats feel their needs are insignificant compared to those of the Ailey Cat. Some Care Cats can be overly self-sacrificing as a way of demonstrating how much they care about the Ailey Cat. Some Care Cats have a hard time giving up control. Some Care Cats want to protect others from having to experience illness and suffering.

The truth is that the needs of Care Cats are just as important as those of the Ailey Cat. When Care Cats assume an unsustainable amount of responsibility, they risk burning out. It can be hard to reconcile, in the face of endless care needs, that your number-one priority is to take care of yourself, but if you burn out, you won't be able to help your Ailey Cat at all and may risk becoming ill yourself.

Do a wellness check with yourself every day. Be honest about whether you are getting enough sleep, eating enough, drinking enough water, exercising, and taking breathers to enjoy some time off duty. If not, reevaluate your situation. Review the tips in this section for ideas on how to take care of yourself.

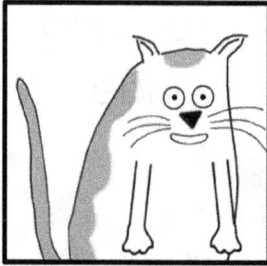
Primary Care Cat

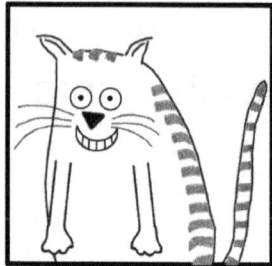
Backup Cat, relieves
Primary Care Cat

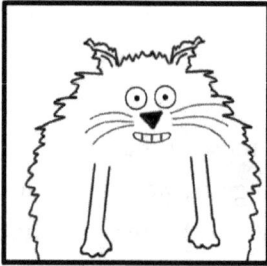
Admin Cat, tracks info on
spreadsheet

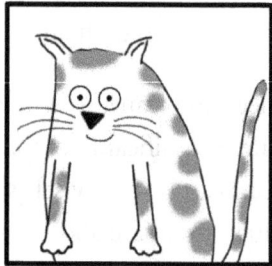
Advocate Cat, goes to all
doctor appointments

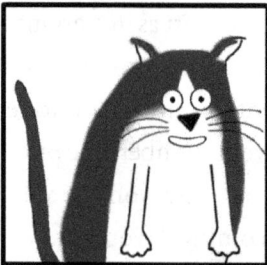
Comm Cat, handles
communications and organizes
volunteers

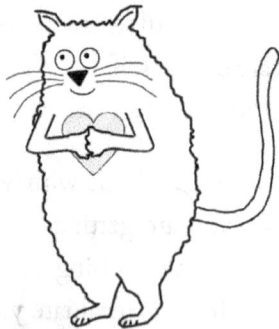
Grateful Ailey Cat

Recognize That Caregiving Requires a Team

For Ailey Cats who require a high level of care, it's essential to have a team so that the responsibility doesn't fall to one person. Having a team also helps keep Care Cats in the game through mutual support and camaraderie.

Assembling a caregiving team can be challenging. People have busy lives. Professional home care can be expensive. Ailey Cats may feel vulnerable and resist having people they don't know in their living space. Ailey Cats may not have many (or any) support people.

You may need to reach out to hospital social workers, local faith communities, neighborhood groups, or local support services (for example, hospice or organizations that provide meals or rides to appointments). Websites of national or local caregiver organizations may also have useful resources.

If you have enough people to form a team, it can be helpful to assign specific roles so each person is clear on how they will be helping. There are some excellent (and usually free) online scheduling and communication tools you can use to keep everyone in the loop.

Seek out a therapist, support group, or trusted friends

Join an online caregiver group

Explore stress-reduction strategies such as mindfulness meditation, 4-7-8 breathing, 61-points relaxation body scan, or Emotional Freedom Technique

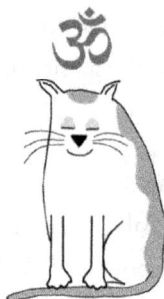

Write in a journal

Take a nap

Take a walk

Go for a drive

Rub your feet

Rub your ribs

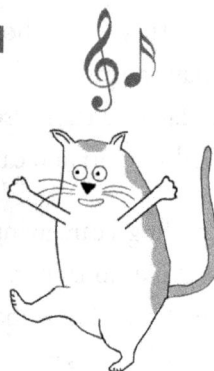

Put on some music and dance

Do some stretches

Take a bath with Epsom salts

Go to a restaurant where you're waited on

Get a massage or other bodywork

Get a microwavable bean bag neck warmer

Most important: Recruit help— see "Recognize That Caregiving Requires a Team")

Be Your Own Care Cat

To take good care of an Ailey Cat who requires a high level of care, you must take care of yourself. There may seem to be an unending list of things to handle for your Ailey Cat, and it may feel impossible to step away to tend to your own needs. But if you don't, you risk burning out. If you collapse, you won't be able to help your Ailey Cat. Keep in mind that sometimes even a seemingly small bit of self-care can go a long way.

If you aren't the primary Care Cat, you can still be of great help by:

- Reminding the primary Care Cat of the necessity of self-care, and that one person can only do so much

- Acknowledging what they're going through, being a witness and a sounding board

- Encouraging them to take breathers, such as, "We're going for a bike ride"

- Filling in while they step away (or contributing money to hire additional help)

- Gifting them a massage, restaurant gift card, or other self-care activities

- Just being there to keep them company—caregiving can get lonely

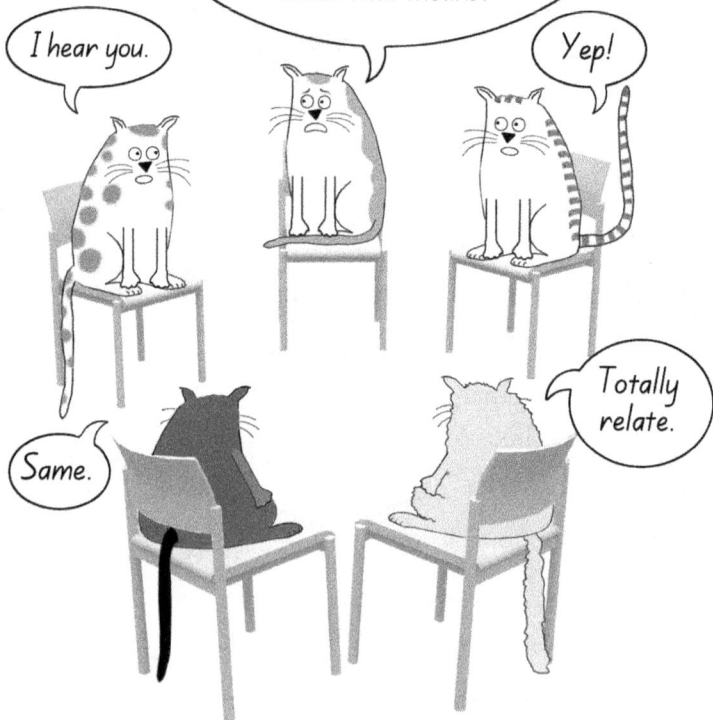

Taking Care of Yourself When Dealing with a Difficult Cat

Sometimes an Ailey Cat isn't their best self and they take their frustration out on their Care Cats. It can be especially challenging if an Ailey Cat is always difficult—it's important to acknowledge that not all care relationships are harmonious!

While there is no easy answer, these strategies may be helpful:

- Don't go it alone—engage others to give you some time away.

- Find a way to discharge your frustrations, such as through exercising, journaling, or talking to a therapist, trusted friend, or support group.

- Think about the underlying source of their behavior and know that it's not personal.

- Try to defuse the situation by:

  - Validating their feelings: "Did it feel like things were out of control?"

  - Putting a hand on their arm and gently asking, "Are you having a hard time right now?"

  - Reminding them, "I'm on your side."

  - Setting a gentle boundary: "I love you, but things affect me, too. I need you to stop yelling at me."

- If it happens only occasionally, think of their behavior as weather that comes and goes, but isn't who they are.

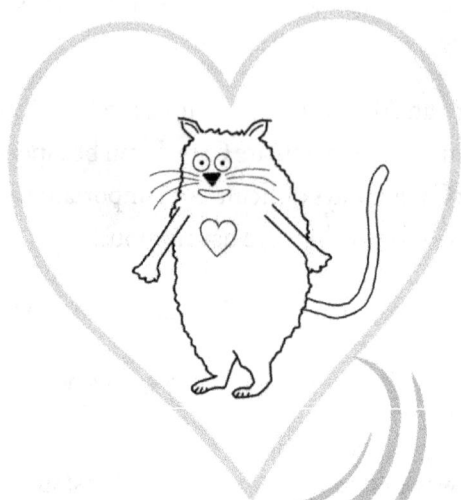

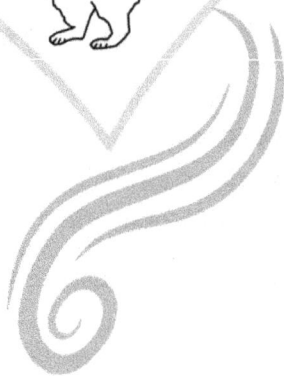

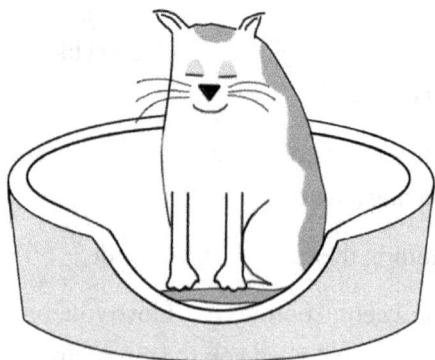

Hold Light Instead of Worrying

It may be impossible not to worry about your Ailey Cat, and at times the worry can feel all-consuming. It's heartbreaking to feel as if there is nothing more you can do to help your Ailey Cat.

In those moments, this practice of "holding light" for your Ailey Cat may help:

1. Find a comfortable, quiet place to sit or lie down.

2. Tune into your breathing.

3. Take some deep breaths.

4. Open to the feeling, or resonance, of light as a positive sense of goodness, grace, kindness, generosity, compassion, faith, devotion, deep acceptance, love. Take whatever time you need to breathe this particular virtue of feeling into your heart and through your body.

5. Think about your Ailey Cat. See them in your mind's eye, breathe deeply, and radiate that light to them. Do this for as long as feels right to you.

Doing this exercise puts you in an *active* state, in which you are sending good energy to your Ailey Cat, rather than a *passive* state of worry. It can be a powerful antidote to feeling collapsed or stuck in trouble or concern. No matter the outcome, holding light is good for both you and your Ailey Cat, and it's something that can be practiced at any time.

A Quick List of Things to Say and Not Say

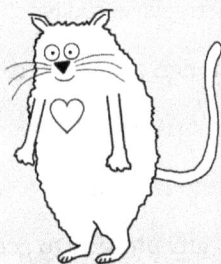

Helpful

- I've been thinking about you.

- It's nice to see you.

- How are you today?

- This is really hard.

- I hate that you got bad news, I'm sorry.

- I'm sorry you have to go through this.

- I hear you, it's terrible.

- How is your energy level today?

- Do you have enough energy for that today?

- What level is your pain at today?

- How did you sleep last night?

- Please don't feel any pressure to get back to me right away.

- I just wanted to let you know I'm thinking of you.

- It's not fair, it sucks, I'm sorry.

- I'm sorry, that was insensitive of me.

- I don't know what to say, but I'm sad for you.

- You've been on my mind. I'm hoping you're okay even though I know you're not okay.

- I don't know what to say, I'm just so sorry.

- I heard you were having health issues, I'm really sorry.

- If you want to tell me more about what's going on for you, I'm here to listen.

- You're dealing with so much.

- You're going through a really difficult passage and doing the best you can; remember to be gentle with yourself.

- It seems like you're having a totally natural response to awful circumstances.

- How is that for you?

- Do you want to tell me more?

- Would you like to set up a time to get together and talk more?

- I'd like to come and help you with a project. If you're ready, let's get something on the calendar.

Not Helpful

- How long do you have?
- How long do people with your health condition usually live?
- I heard it was psychological.
- Seems like everyone has [whatever your Ailey Cat has] these days.
- Does this affect your sex life?
- You're going to be okay, I know it!
- I know how you feel.
- You're too young for this.
- You should be better by now.
- Keep me posted!
- Let me know if you need anything.
- Have you tried _____?
- You need to try _____.
- You should _____.
- Just push through it!
- My best friend's ex-brother-in-law had the same thing.
- If you just [ate better/exercised more/lost weight] you'd be better.
- You're sick because _____.

- Everyone gets tired.
- Everyone gets aches and pains.
- But you don't look sick.
- Aren't you worried about the side effects of the medications you're taking?
- You're too young to have aching joints.
- I wish I had what you have, then maybe I could lose weight.
- This is your new normal.
- You'll get used to it.
- This, too, shall pass.
- Everything works out in the end.
- You'll be there for [some future event]!
- It's only hair, it will grow back.
- You'll have new, perky boobs!
- Oh, you poor thing!
- You're going to win this battle, you're a strong warrior!
- This will make you a stronger person.
- Look on the bright side…
- Stay positive!
- Don't think that way!
- You look so different!
- You have an excuse to stay in bed and sleep.

- There is always a gift in great pain.

- Everything happens for a reason.

- What doesn't kill you makes you stronger.

- It could be worse.

- It is what it is.

- At least you don't have _____.

- You can never be too rich or too thin.

- We all could die at any moment.

- Don't worry, God will heal you.

- It's God's plan.

- Life only gives you what you can handle.

About The Author

Sheila Hoover has a PhD in Adult Education and over twenty years of experience making content accessible for audiences in creative and engaging ways. She is also the author of *Helping Through Heartache: An Easy Guide to Supporting Anyone Who is Grieving*. She has trained and practiced as an end-of-life doula, supporting friends and family with serious illnesses and chronic health conditions.

www.ingramcontent.com/pod-product-compliance
Lightning Source LLC
Chambersburg PA
CBHW060459280326
41933CB00014B/2797